For Paul and Helen

Contents

Preface

This book was born of a double wish: to understand our cultural preoccupation with the skin and to explore the newly emerged scientific knowledge of how it works. My own scientific career was steeped in skin biology. I learned how to produce tumors in the skin of mice in record time (three weeks) and how to help the body control what happens to those tumors. Doing this work, I made thousands of skin grafts. I studied how the body's immune system learns to recognize foreignness. I studied hundreds of histological preparations of the skin to see how it looked under the microscope. And in 1968 I discovered that sometimes the immune system could march all the way to the skin's surface to rein in a blossoming skin tumor, the first demonstration of immune surveillance in the newly appreciated field of tumor immunology.

In writing this book, I wanted to go beyond the simple biology of the skin to explore how we define our "edge," or boundary with the outer world. It is unclear just how we learn as infants to monitor where we stop and the world begins. What are the origins of the expressions "thin-skinned" or "thick-skinned"? Do they have a biological basis? How is it that new schools of psychotherapy treat the skin as a literal extension of our inner selves and use tactile relearning as a basis for therapy? How do we use the skin to advertise ourselves, and how does society treat those who through no fault of their own display the cutaneous stigmata of disease or illness?

The skin can be a biological neon sign, advertising our race, health, and mental state. Not long ago, the purple splotches of Kaposi's sarcoma, a hallmark of AIDS, were the equivalent of Hester Prynne's red *A* in Hawthorne's *Scarlet Letter*. Individuals with Kaposi's were socially ostracized. For some people, a mass of tattoos is one statement of individuality, while the scars of self-mutilation—or suicide attempts—denote another.

Former cultures invested heavily in the skin's symbolic importance. Greek mythology treated the skin as a trophy, a shield, or a vulnerable membrane. Medusa's look could turn skin to stone. Native American cultures considered the possession of someone's skin (a scalp) the ultimate declaration of vindication of an enemy. Why is the skin so heavily vested with symbolic importance?

Eastern schools of medicine treated the skin as a literal mirror of our inner wellness. Diagnoses were made from a glance at skin color, rashes, or spots. For the Chinese, nuanced changes in the skin and tongue sufficed for diagnoses.

In contrast, Western medical practitioners are often stymied by the diverse signs on the skin that denote internal illness. At one time, when the body turned against itself in autoimmune diseases like lupus erythematosus or in the cutaneous form of tuberculosis, physicians foolishly treated the skin problem as if it were the whole disease. We now know that the butterfly rash across the nose and cheeks that characterizes lupus or the skin signs of TB are symptomatic of attacks throughout the organism. Why did we so often stop our ministrations at the surface of the body?

Pharmaceutical and cosmetic companies vie with each other to develop more and better nostrums for the skin. Like the Conquistadors' quest for the mythical El Dorado, the Aztec man of gold-skin, their searches and discoveries are part fanciful and part real. Some, like silicone injections, engendered false hopes of a permanent and innocuous cure for aging. Others are bona fide scientific accomplishments, such as collagen and vitamin A analogs that can encourage regeneration of dermal tissues. But where are the roots of this obsession grounded, and why are so many worthless remedies still permitted on the market?

Behind the obsession with new cosmetic products is a powerful motivation. Consumers spend more money on the skin than any other health condition, pouring billions of dollars annually into questionable remedies like jojoba oil and herbal antioxidants or on drugs with potent and dangerous properties like tretinoin or its analog, Retin-A. Even as the environmental damage from chemical carcinogens and the depletion of the ozone layer become more certain, medical practitioners continue to advocate passive protection (sunscreens), while governments concede only minor reductions in their production of halogenated ozone depleters. In the meantime, DNA-damaging ultraviolet light continues to pour inexorably at ever-increasing levels onto the earth's surface. Over the next decades, what will be the consequences to our most vulnerable outer membrane of this industrial excess?

Sun seekers still vie with each other to get the "best" tan, and medical treatments for some of the more serious diseases like psoriasis rely on ultraviolet light, a known carcinogen. Just how does society balance the risks and benefits of all the factors that come into play? Our skin is often the litmus test and the slate on which these stories are told.

Acknowledgments

This book could not have been written without the support of my spouse and children. I thank them profusely. Also, thanks to Cynthia Vartan of Henry Holt and Company for her diligent editing and her confidence in my abilities. Thanks also to Albert Rosenfeld for sharing his own earlier articles on the skin, and to Dr. Gerald Donnelly, who first showed me the ravages of basal cell carcinoma and thereby whetted my appetite for more knowledge about the skin. Special thanks to Gordon Smith, CMT, who helped me understand the roots of beneficial massage.

ONE

Introduction
to the Integument

The skin is much more than a pallid canvas of beauty or the passive interface between ourselves and a hostile environment. Our skin serves as a real and metaphoric boundary between ourselves and others, between health and disease.

Our own self-images often unconsciously incorporate the skin metaphors of our lives. When we look in the mirror, few of us think of our skin as the resilient, protective sheath that shields us from an often inimical environment. We see it instead in all its imagined frailty, a highly vulnerable organ that tears or bleeds at the slightest cut. Many of us picture ourselves as "thin-skinned," subject to the vagaries of a hostile world. Our attitude toward our skin is revealed in the way we treat it. We hide and color it, abrade and reshape it, dissatisfied at our natural lot. Sometimes we are so ashamed of our natural visage that we abuse it, resorting to cosmetic surgery to "fix" it or piercing lips or tongue to vaunt it.

We are unique in the animal world in that the configuration of skin on our faces reveals every emotion or feeling. When locked in to a single expression, it armors us against emotional threats from others. When relaxed and open to our emotional selves, it is a marvelous organ of expression and feeling. The best thespians and directors know that to mold the exterior self to the interior feelings is a sublime art, one that requires the most direct communication between the soul and the innervation that controls the twenty-four muscles of the face.

Over time, the most used muscles and thence the most experienced emotions become etched in the lines of our faces. Montaigne once said that by the age of thirty-five we are responsible for our face. Members of preliterate societies recognized this fact and regarded the skin as a tableau of a life. The faces of Geronimo and Sitting Bull still paint a picture to some of us of great suffering and nobility. We grant faint tribute to these marks of courage or weakness as "character lines." But in other cultures at other times, facial lines carried immense symbolic value. An Australian aborigine teenage boy was once more drawn to the wizened face of an elder woman of the tribe than to any fresh-faced young female. In Western society we venerate the tabula rasa of the youthful countenance and abhor wrinkles.

In spite of our best efforts to stymie its natural course, all facial skin progresses inexorably to a wizened, wrinkled, and blemished state. While much of this decay is an inevitable consequence of biology, most of the visible signs of aging are the result of environmental exposure. Being at the forefront of our battle with the environment, the skin is often the first to flag and suffer. Natural forces of wind, cold, and sunlight waste it.

As we age, so does our skin, through failing replenishment and ultimate accelerated death. Would we do better at accepting its passage if we knew that our skin is always dying? Our skin dies a little every day—and replenishes itself at the same time. Like the grass that the Egyptian pharaohs used in the *Book of the Dead*, the ever-replenishing skin is a metaphor for resurrection. Have we somehow forgotten that life's struggle against entropy is acted out on our bodies? From embryogenesis on, little islands of new cells appear, wax, and wane in our skin. First genetic instructions and later chemicals or sunlight shape their evolution from pigmented freckles to malignant nevi, from limpid pools of translucent beauty to the "horrid brown spots" of old age. Our skin passes from a childhood mirror of beauty to the wizened keratoses of old age as certainly as day begets night. And still we struggle against it.

If beauty depends on achieving youthful-appearing skin, the sun is its nemesis. The same sunlight that gives us that Hollywood-inspired bronzed vigor produces cancer. Every modern-day model knows that sunlight is anathema to beauty. It is one of the greatest ironies of our times that the same chemicals that permitted the cosmetic products of the 1960s and 1970s to be sprayed from cans gave us a depleted ozone layer that contributes to skin aging. Ozone depletion adds tremendously to the burden of high-energy ultraviolet radiation that is almost certainly linked to the growing epidemic of solar-associated skin cancer in Australia. Could any Greek god conceive of a more divine justice to the daily reliance of developed countries on aerosolized perfumes, hairsprays, and deodorants than disfiguring skin cancer?

Through a Mirror Darkly

In Ancient cultures, the skin once held a higher place than it does today. The skin was once regarded as a vulnerable portal to the body through which both good and evil influences could penetrate. When the body needed medication, drugs and poultices were spread on the skin. As described in the Ebers Papyrus, one of the first two medical treatises known from ancient Egypt, pastes of various fats, honey, natron, salt, dough, and yeasts were applied to the skin to treat illness lodged in the stomach or other internal organs.[1] Shamans of the Yanomami Indians of the Amazon who wished to influence the course of disease would blow herb-rich smoke over a victim's body, to be absorbed by the skin. Similarly, Yagu shamans of Peru blow the smoke from a large cigar over their own bodies to "soften" the skin so that they may later release therapeutic "darts" from within their bodies. The shaman throws these "darts" at a sleeping patient, often making cures all the more miraculous because the unconscious patient is unaware of his treatment, thus belying the Western assumption that all such ministrations work through a placebo effect.

The taboo against breaching the skin either in life or death was so strong in other societies, notably the Chinese, that neither autopsy nor hypodermic needles evolved. In ancient China, the skin was seen as an external manifestation of the inner workings of the body, a place where diagnosis could be made by examining that extension of our skin, the tongue, or palpating the three pulses. Treatments followed external "meridians" along the body's surface that represented inner organs and penetrated them at critical junctures known as acupuncture points.

Today, all this has been changed. We are preoccupied with the expressionless, smooth skin of our models. Cindy Crawford's fawnlike skin is captured in a full body shot on the cover of my current issue of *Esquire* magazine under the banner WOMEN WE LOVE. For Cindy "wannabes," cosmetic companies offer literally a dozen ads inside its cover that promise instant beauty. Hundreds of new and often only transiently effective medications to keep skin looking young are put on the market each year. In the mid-1990s, botanicals offer the greatest allure. Whole new lines of cosmetics, like those from a local California firm called Garden Botanika, promise natural remedies to the normal vagaries of skin that wax and wane with the menstrual cycle or dissipate with old age.

Historically, skin-deep beauty was often achieved at the expense of the body as a whole. The Ebers Papyrus contains passages that describe in great detail cosmetics such as hair colorants, eyeliners, rouge, and lipsticks. Some, like the eyeliners based on lead salts, continued to be used through Greek and Roman times and were undoubtedly dangerous and possibly toxic. Later, in the Middle Ages and through the Renaissance, arsenic was used as a skin treatment to cause a blush to appear on the cheeks, even though absorption of this potent poison would likely have damaged the bone marrow and produced anemia.

Although the remarkable permeability of the skin that makes these superficial ministrations so dangerous was recognized by nineteenth-century physicians, occupational and environmental risks from skin-absorbed toxins were virtually ignored until recently. In the 1970s hundreds of workers experienced contact dermatitis and systemic poisoning from pesticides like malathion that were readily absorbed through the skin. While many dermatology professionals now recognize the crucial importance of skin permeation in preventive medicine, drug companies have capitalized on skin permeability for cosmetic or relatively trivial medical ends. Thousands of drug delivery creams and skin patches of such questionable nostrums as antioxidants, "natural" progesterone, nicotine, and caffeine have been marketed in the last decade. Others, including skin-delivered heart and blood pressure medications, are still being evaluated. As I show in chapter 5, even such seemingly valuable drugs as nitroglycerin lose their potency after being delivered day after day through the skin.

Belief Origins

The roots of our cultural preoccupation with the skin presage a number of our modern medical mistakes. Many of our beliefs about the skin are imbued with superstition and myth. In ancient Greece, skin color alone was deemed the most reliable marker of bodily well-being. Among the most far-reaching Greek ideas, the concept of the four humors was embraced en bloc by virtually all medical practitioners through the Renaissance and into the eighteenth century. Galen, who developed this theoretical construct after the works of Hippocrates, wrote about the theory in the second century A.D. According to Galen, there are four humors in the human body: blood, phlegm, and two biles, black and yellow. If these humors are balanced, a person is healthy; if imbalanced, he or she is sick. In medieval times physicians relied on often mistaken readings of Greek medicine, believing that the complexion alone could be used to diagnose the state of these four elements in the body.[2] With the Renaissance and the appearance of the great anatomist and medical illustrator Andreas Vesalius (1514– 1564), true diagnosis of organ-specific disease emerged, and the skin as a diagnostic tool took a backseat to more formal rules of the analysis of disease.

While many diseases provide ample clues to their pathogenesis in skin changes (explored in depth in chapter 6), physicians today commonly overlook the skin in developing their diagnostic impressions. As the author of the chapter on skin diseases in the most authoritative modern medical text, the *Cecil Textbook of Medicine*, observes, "The student attuned to palpating and auscultating [listening as with a stethoscope] forgets to look. He misses basic physiologic facts about his patient, perhaps significant signals of serious disease. Further, when the patient draws attention to a skin change, the student is uncertain as to what it may be or its importance."[3]

The Skin as Barrier

An almost universal sense of human frailty in the face of the elements is reflected in our attitudes toward the skin. We perceive our skin as if it were only a physical barrier between ourselves and a hostile world.

The view of the skin as a barrier against pathogens, pollutants, and radiation is a modern one, and a wrong-headed one at that. Many primitive cultures regarded the skin as a naturally permeable system and respected its integrity by limiting their disinfection efforts to occasional scrubbings. As I will document in chapter 3, modern medical practitioners mistakenly believe that the skin must be kept "clean" and germ-free as a defense against disease. Through the overzealous use of disinfectants, the skin is stripped of its naturally protective microorganisms. This unfortunate practice has led to nursery epidemics of antibiotic-resistant staph and streptococcal skin infections and overgrowth of yeast organisms. Misplaced efforts to prevent the normal seeding of a newborn's skin with a mother's natural bacteria—commonly transferred in breast-feeding—is one cause of these disasters. Overreliance on antibiotics or hormones to control infection of the skin by acne-producing bacteria is another. Acne itself spawned a whole industry of cosmetics and drugs, with sometimes disastrous consequences.

Indeed, the profound emotional reaction to what is otherwise a self-limiting and nonfatal condition spawned an intense competition to find powerful acne-limiting drugs. The *Physicians' Desk Reference* lists thirty-five different prescription drugs that are marketed in the United States for this use alone. One of these "success" stories led to the second greatest birth defect disaster (after thalidomide) in our time. The story of Accutane, the only drug found to control cystic acne, is told in chapter 6.

A similar preoccupation colors our efforts at controlling skin aging. The attempt to replace or repair age- or disease-damaged skin has also been a perennial quest of medicine. Like the antiacne medications, today's inventions, including collagen, silicone, antioxidants, and artificial membranes, are fraught with problems as well as promise. The story of these developments is one of often premature and misguided attempts to fill a culturally dictated need to retain youthfulness, if not beauty, into old age.

Obsession with Skin

Of all of the attributes associated with the skin, it is the ineffable one of beauty that puts the skin at the center of our lives. The culture of beauty that transfixes Americans turns on maintaining an irrationally nubile appearance of our skin. In the words of a leading skin product company, "Western society's view of beauty [is] based on young, smooth, wrinkle-free skin—an ideal perpetuated by the mainstream cosmetics industry."[4] The impossible dream of eternally youthful, "perfect" skin is an invention of this industry, even as it encourages activities like suntanning, chemical "peels," and dermabrasion that are inimical to the skin's survival in its youthful form.

Faces

Perhaps more than any other element that fuels the persistent obsession with our skin's appearance is the psychic energy we have invested in maintaining a youthful, often expressionless visage. In doing so, we sometimes forget that the face is the screen on which our individual life drama is acted out. We learn to recognize its distinguishing features as newborn infants. As adults we can pick out a familiar face from a photomontage of literally thousands of strangers. Instead of cherishing its uniqueness, people expend fortunes to mold the face into a banal simulacrum. They permit it to be reshaped, injected, and stretched until it loses its distinctive character, sometimes erasing generations of genetic and ethnic selection with a single cut.

In the movie *The Mask*, "putting on a new face" becomes a metaphor for our time. The premise is simple: A meek soul played by actor Jim Carrey discovers an elastic face mask that can bend and shape with his every whim. This new face transforms him into a self-assertive, attractive "wise guy." Ironically, just a decade earlier, a movie with the same name (*Mask*) told a different story. Here a young boy afflicted with neurofibromatosis, the disease that crippled the Elephant Man, must go through life burdened by the stigma of a monstrous-looking face he cannot change. His triumph is achieving his own humanity and individuality with the aid of his mother. But throughout his short life, his wish to change his appearance, illustrated by a fantasy sequence of his looking in a distorting mirror at an amusement park, dominates his psyche. For any child with this disease, such a wish is more than understandable. But for many of us fortunate to have normal features, the modern quest to reshape ourselves through makeup or cosmetic surgery has become an unhealthy obsession.

Our culture perpetuates the myth of metamorphosis—that change is possible. If we could change our skin like a snake, our lives could be transformed from the mundane to the spectacular. So we imagine how we might look younger, erase the frown lines on our brow, or change our entire visage. This book explores the roots of this obsession and reveals some of the basic truths about the skin. It is both more and less than we make of it, having newfound medical significance even as we discover our limited ability to truly change it.

TWO

At the Boundary of the Self

The skin is both literally and metaphorically "the body's edge." It is what defines our outermost limits and declares our emotions to the outside world. We all recognize the physical signs of our emotional responses: we steel our jaw, set our faces, and tighten the skin around our mouths when we want to appear tough. Our lips curl, our hair stands up, and the skin around our eyes widens when we are fearful.

Our sense of psychic well-being is inextricably linked with our skin. The skin provides our psyches with a metaphor for protection, a boundary against an inimical world. Being thick-skinned is "good," as if resistance to emotions were bound up with this protective barrier. Who has not talked about an annoying work partner "getting under my skin"? By the same token, we speak about someone we love in the same way. (Remember the lyrics to "I've Got You Under My Skin"?)

In a strange way, we identify our skin with our innermost selves. We talk about wishing to "change our skin" when what we are really after is a total psychic overhaul. We use skin metaphors to describe our relationships. An easily rattled character is called "thin-skinned." Someone who is readily turned on sensually is said to have "highly responsive skin." Being "in touch" with someone today is not simply a physical statement.

The skin is in fact a metaphor for much of our contemporary psychic uneasiness. We are "out of touch" with reality, armored against feelings, and insensitive to others. In truth, we *don't* want anyone "getting under our skin."

All of us recognize the palpable discomfort that comes from unwanted touching. But consider for a moment the possibility that the vague sense of personal uneasiness many of us feel in a crowd may also have a biological basis. Is it possible that we not only pick up subliminal cues from the expressions or body postures of others, but that we have lost some deeper, cutaneous sensibility to our surroundings? Many neurophysiologists are convinced that humans are literally less sensitive to external reality than are other mammals. Our nerve endings are less dense than those of other mammals, many of whom rely on their skin and sense of touch for survival. Some nocturnal animals like the raccoon have extraordinary senses of touch, allowing them to feel out underwater prey or distinguish edible food from garbage.

We also know that the skin once played a much larger role in sensing the environment. We know of fish who sense their environment almost entirely through their skin, using a lateral line system to pick up vibrations through the water. Electric eels project a force field around themselves and then sense the response cutaneously.

Perhaps agoraphobia—a fear of crowds—and our cultural tendency toward "insensitivity" have biological roots in these physiological realities. Was it once adaptive to "feel" the presence of strangers? Were we always so cutaneously unaware of our surroundings? Like cave fish who have lost their sense of sight, humankind may have lost a richer sense of touch that is no longer needed. It is tempting to speculate that a heightened sense of external awareness, once mediated through our skin, has been lost only recently, leaving behind just a vague sense of "personal space."

This hypothesized diminution of cutaneous sensibility may be an evolutionary consequence of our almost exclusive reliance on our primary senses. With the dominance of sight, and to a lesser extent hearing and smell, almost all of our attention has been concentrated on our brain's newest structures, its cortical regions. If our peripheral sensory systems have been understimulated and underused in recent evolutionary time, any associated sensory apparatus would have languished.

Primates and humans in particular are distinguished from other groups of higher animals in having almost all of their contact to the outside world concentrated in their central sensorium: the eyes, nose, and mouth. When once an infant handled an object, now it "mouths" it. The resulting reinforcement of reliance on the cranial nerves and associated cortical centers in the brain may have caused what evolutionists speak of as "relaxed natural selection." As a result of disuse, our peripheral nervous system became less richly innervated (supplied with nerves). Without the constant reinforcement of skin sensation, the selective pressures that once favored highly nerve-rich, skin-sensitive individuals may have given way to those that favor individuals with highly centralized processing abilities—and blunted skin sensibility. Through disuse we may have lost one of our most critical contacts with the outside world.

Occasional experiments of nature point to the fact that this "loss" may be real. A few rare humans who "feel" deeply have come to do so by intensifying their abilities to feel "superficially." By all accounts Helen Keller, deprived shortly after birth of sight and sound, was one of the most humane and sensitive individuals of the twentieth century. Keller's ability to call on residual sensory systems, especially in her fingertips, that measure vibration, touch, and pressure may have contributed to her humanity. If so, then the ability to become fully human through reinforcement of the cutaneous pathways is a route open to all of us. Our loss of contact with our surroundings is recoverable: Keller's triumph shows that it is more a reversible developmental process than a permanent loss.

Wearing clothes may restrict the full development of sensory abilities by walling us off still further from critical skin sensory contact, especially as children. Our cultural insistence on oral and written communication over the more tactile arts may further limit those with a human skin that is highly innervated. Only those few who, like Erick Hawkins or Nijinsky, find a medium where sensory stimulation is paramount may rescue their sensoria from the tyranny of visual dominance.

If ontogeny really does recapitulate phylogeny by taking embryos through more primitive-appearing forms, we might expect to see vestiges of this more highly innervated, ultrasensitive individual in the process of embryogenesis. Indeed, some infants born prematurely often have such excruciating hypersensitivity to tactile stimuli that they cannot stand being touched. Their irritability may be a result of the immaturity of their peripheral and central nervous systems.

Only later, at full term, is the newborn infant capable of accepting the skin contact that is so essential a part of the maternal-infant bond. For many of us who did not have this bonding through an intense nursing period, the psychic loss may be lifelong. Maintaining the constant skin contact and pressure of the uterus in the immediate postpartum period may also be critical for optimal development, a reality underscored by the commonness of swaddling among diverse cultures.

Later in childhood, skin contact appears to lose its primacy as a means of communication and linkage with others. There may be a biological basis for this transition. Certain changes in innervation during ontogeny provide a clue to the loss of the primacy of the skin as a major sensorium. Early in embryogenesis, the peripheral nervous system is highly vulnerable and virtually naked: little or no myelin insulation covers the peripheral nerves that course along the blood vessels of the developing fetus to the limbs and skin surface. After myelination has caught up with the peripheral motor and sensory nerves at about two years, some nerves apparently "die back," reducing the richness of innervation of the skin. After loss of high-frequency vibration hearing, tactile sensitivity also declines with age, reflecting the lack of reserve of the skin's neurosensory apparatus.

While anatomists often emphasize how well endowed human skin is with nerve endings, they often overlook the fact that such rich innervation is highly limited. Only on the ends of our fingers and in our few remaining erogenous zones are there sufficient densities of nerves to respond to subtle stimuli.

Denervation

It is a profound paradox of nature that the boundary where we leave off and our external environment begins is demarcated by an organ with so few sensory systems and nerves. With the exception of creatures that are literally "armored," like the arthropods and Insecta generally, no other organism in our phylum has so few contacts with the outer world. (An exception may be the armored armadillo, which has only a few sensory hairs that transect its body armor to bring it cutaneous awareness of its physical surroundings.) For most members of the mammalian order, the outer integument is shot through with highly sensitive sensory apparatus designed to detect temperature and humidity changes and the minute vibrations that signal the presence of prey. For *Homo sapiens* this apparent loss of sensory ability has condemned us to a diminished world.

If my hypothesis is correct, over evolution the sensoria that reside in the skin have been blunted as higher centers that co-ordinated visual and auditory cues became more important to survival. Those cutaneous sensory systems that once enabled us to experience a rich and varied world of texture, pressure, heat, and vibration have been dampened and replaced by this more central system.

Today, when we say we "know" what a roar sounds like and means, we are processing the sound through our ears and audi-tory cortex. But the deeper, low-frequency vibratory cues you can still feel faintly in your skin and viscera may have told our ancestors other, more critical information: whether the growl/roar was a threat or a bluff, whether we should fight or flee. In the absence of these cutaneous and visceral cues, all we are left with is a vague sense of uneasiness. Motion picture sound track experts capitalized on this atavistic reaction by en-coding the low-frequency tones into the "shark" music of *Jaws* or the bass-dominant theme of Darth Vader in *Star Wars*. These experts know that when we are bombarded by low-frequency sound waves people feel anxious and fearful. The receptors for picking up these vibrations are still present: some are probably lodged solidly in our skin. But they are few and far between.

Now, instead of feeling force fields, energy, and vibration through our skin, we dully experience only blunt pain, frigid cold, or searing heat. It is clear that the ascendancy of the visual cortex has diminished our reliance on other senses.

A key question that arises from all this is if loss of our cuta-neous sensorium has been so recent that we have failed to pro-vide adequate stimulation to insure normal development. Kinesthesiologists have long recognized that the skin is a portal to physical as well as psychic wellness. Dyslexic children can be taught to read by cutaneous reprogramming, a procedure by which they are allowed to *feel* the shapes of letters with their fingers. Whole schools of psychotherapy are now based on restoring this linkage between the external sensorium and the inner self. Repatterning, in which the skin is systematically stroked and stimulated, is now part of the therapy for autism, and massage is an increasingly valued adjunct to psychotherapy. Transformational therapy relies on skin and deep tissue massage to evoke deep emotional events that are "stored" in the soma or muscles. Massage therapists have been able to help hypersensitive children by providing skin stimuli where sound and sight are overwhelming. The ultimate success of these still experimental forms of therapy appears to depend on restoring the richness of our cutaneous contact with the outer world.

Skin and Sensation

Other evolutionary factors may have accelerated the trend toward withdrawal from cutaneous stimuli. Our need for individual protection from the outside world decreased with the formation of social groups wherein one dominant individual could be the eyes and ears of the troop. Also, the vulnerability brought about by our upright posture and loss of hair literally caused our skins to become thicker, especially among males. As a result, the one system that we rely on to perceive the natural world most intimately—our skin—became covered with a deadened casement. At our surface we are enshrouded by a lining of lifeless tissue, the stratum corneum of the anatomists.

As evidence of this desensitization, there are places on the human back where a person cannot perceive the difference in sensation between two needlepoints held an inch apart and the prick of a needle at a single point. And nerve endings at the base of hair follicles in the skin that once could perceive subtle vibrations now respond only with a "tickle" sensation to direct stimuli. Although we once had hair that would literally stand on end through the action of the pilar erectus muscles, few if any of us today retain sufficient nerve densities even to get the skin on the nape of our neck to stand up when we are terrified. Paradoxically, when people experience a release of stress during massage therapy, some get "gooseflesh" from the action of these same "tenting" muscles on the parts of their bodies being worked.[1]

Deep within the skin itself, pressure-sensitive proprioceptive nerves designed to perceive minute changes in the tension of the skin now record sensations from only blunt pressure and the strongest cutaneous stimuli, while more sensitive receptors are few and far apart (see chapter 3). A few "sensitive" individuals may have retained greater numbers of these latter receptors. Throughout history, individuals have claimed to retain a remarkable vibration sensitivity. John Dillinger, the notorious safecracker, was said to be able to "feel" in his fingertips when the lock tumblers fell into place. But people like Dillinger are exceptions to the general rule of blunted sensory awareness in the skin. Stories from Russia of psychics able to read type through their fingertips have since been debunked. Some of these individuals do appear to have an ability to detect subtle variations in infrared radiation through their fingertips, making "finger reading" a more credible claim. And Kirlian photographs (thus named in 1939 after their Soviet inventor) of faint electric discharges show that a skin force field may be a reality.

Psychological Implications

Most of us are still left with a much impoverished perception of our external world. Many psychiatric disturbances that concern self-image come to be played out at the body's edge, an often muted sensory wasteland between ourselves and the outer world. It is no accident that the language of folklore and psychology alike speaks of "well-armored" or "thick-skinned" individuals who stave off psychological incursions by dampening emotions and creating mental blocks against injuries to the self.

As we saw, where the body's edge is hypersensitive as a result of premature birth, an affected individual may barely stand to be touched. Such hyperaesthenic individuals often experience intense isolation from their bewildered parents. Conversely, when infants are born via cesarean section, they may become "tactically defensive" as children or adolescents. These infants appear to need intense tactile stimulation, favoring strong body contact over simply touching: a cesarean-delivered child will often want to be "bear-hugged" rather than just embraced lightly.

Considering that the skin reacts visibly to emotional stimuli (blushing, blanching, and so on), it is obvious to all that the skin and the psyche are interconnected. Indeed, excessive cutaneous stimulation can be the bane of healthy psychic functioning. Many Eastern religious disciplines emphasize the importance of reducing sensory input to achieve the state of mental stillness needed for meditation and release. Meditation must occur in a setting where all sensory stimuli are reduced, including all tactile sensations to the skin. In artificial environments like so-called samadhi tanks intended to accelerate the process of depersonalization, the person is isolated from skin sensations by a buffering zone of still, body-temperature water. In such environments the mind "creates" a new reality, substituting spontaneous neural firings for the sensory inputs that are artificially suppressed. The resulting hallucinations and out-of-body experiences can be used by adepts to achieve altered states of consciousness.

Other psychiatric phenomena are also played out on the

skin. Individuals who go through withdrawal from drug or alcohol addiction feel as if their skin is literally crawling with bugs. This syndrome also occurs among nonaddicted but neurotic persons. It is so common in certain psychiatric circles that it has been given its own name: delusional parasitosis. In this delusional state, the affected persons are convinced that they are infested with parasites; so convinced are they of the reality of their ailment that they often first seek help from dermatologists and not psychiatrists. Some patients even bring in skin scrapings to show the doctor the imagined insects. These samples are almost always devoid of insect remains, although a few persons with scabies have a bona fide disorder that often mimics the delusional one.

Rather than explore the rich symbolic significance of such obsessions, as might have been done by Jung or Freud, modern-day psychiatrists have medicalized the problem. Obsessive disorders that involve the skin are considered metabolic disturbances and are commonly treated with drugs. A typical medication is an antipsychotic agent called pimozide. While it clearly suppresses symptoms, it has severe side effects. Relapses are the rule after discontinuation of the drug.[2]

Dermatology and Psychiatry

The skin itself is also a common target of deep-seated psychoses and neuroses. This is so not simply because it is "reachable," but because of the deep roots that connect a sense of self to the sensorium. For some of us, the skin becomes a focus for obsessive preoccupation. Many individuals struggle with a literal inability to "sense" the self. With the exception of vague proprioceptive sensations that are generated by the intestine and some viscera, the only place where the mind can sense the body is through the skin. This reality often makes the skin the primary canvas on which our cultural and personal identity is drawn.

Given this focus, it is surprising how few linkages exist between dermatology and psychiatry. At least one center exists abroad where the interplay of the psyche and the skin is given top priority. In Ghent, Belgium, there has existed for almost a decade a Department of Psychiatry and Psychodermatology, where particular attention is focused on the neuroses and obsessive disorders. In the United States, only Stanford University and the University of California have formal programs that investigate the mind-body linkage. The Stanford Medical Center has a Dermatology-Psychiatry Liaison Clinic that treats patients for psychiatric disorders and their skin manifestations.

The two pioneers of this work, dermatologist William Gould and psychiatrist Thomas Gragg at the medical center, recognize that the skin can be a magnet for hidden psychological problems. One sign of this relationship is persistent skin lesions that recur regularly. Dr. Gragg has observed, "We see people of all ages, some whose lives appear to be perfectly together. But often they will have delusions about their skin, or skin disorders that don't respond to the usual treatment."[3]

But something deeper is afoot during these dermatopsychiatric disorders. Skin sensations like those experienced in delusional parasitosis are apparently so unsettling that those experiencing them degenerate rapidly into psychosis. What this process may be telling us is that unfamiliar sensory stimuli coming from the skin can be profoundly disturbing.

As any adolescent knows, even mild psychological stress can produce skin disorders, such as acne, or accentuate others, such as psoriasis. Conditions like dermatitis artefacta, in which the skin breaks out in rashes for no apparent reason, or skin hypochondriasis, where patients think their skin is "diseased" when it is not, are described as simple psychosomatic illnesses.[4] They are not.

These textbook descriptions of mild forms of neuroses ignore their progression and hint at the existence of a new and larger group of dermatopsychological disorders. American psychiatry appears to be lagging far behind its European counterparts in understanding the full gamut of meanings associated with self-inflicted acts on the skin. As reflected in the scientific literature, American medicine appears preoccupied with the purely surface implications of skin mutilation, emphasizing physical impairment over mental distress, while others, notably the Scandinavians, have actively described the psychic connections between the skin and the mind.

American physicians often describe the self-mutilating patients they see as being surprised about the severity of the injuries they have inflicted on themselves but go no further in their analysis. An example is the textbook *Dermatological Signs of Internal Disease*, which describes such patients as being unaware of what they have done. Such a view overlooks denial as an important psychological signal and trivializes the deeper causes of cutaneous injury. The authors provide a single provocative note, stating that "the act of producing cutaneous lesions may help the patient define the boundaries of the 'self. . . .' "[5]

Like other dermatology texts, this one stresses the medical cause of injury, emphasizing the damage done by chronic and obsessive scratching and picking to insect bites and local areas of irritation. Such compulsive behaviors are medicalized as simple manifestations of a deficiency in a key neurotransmitter (such as serotonin) or are handled as atypical problems of skin infection control. In either case, the professional treatment of dysfunctional skin behaviors appears to be lacking in appreciation of the psychogenic complexities of self-mutilation generally.

A Case Study of Self-Mutilation

Both psychiatry and dermatology have been caught flat-footed by obsessive disorders such as compulsive hand washing. These problems are emblematic of repetitive, uncontrollable acts that often have deep-seated psychological underpinnings. In the case of a mildly retarded twenty-three-year-old woman who repeatedly wounded her hands and forearms by smashing them against table edges, the psychiatric component of her disorder appears to have been neglected. According to her physician, she was aware that she did this damage when she was under stress. As evidence of her rationality, she had recently changed rooms at home to try to minimize the places where she could hurt herself. She still could not keep the behavior under control, however, and it escalated to full-blown self-mutilation. In spite of evidence of psychological dysfunction, her doctors dismissed her problem as a simple manifestation of poor coping skills. The attending psychiatrist determined that she was "frustrated" by her life. To treat this frustration, he recommended a job change and prescribed medication to dampen her anxieties.[6] Without second-guessing her physicians' interventions, I suspect this diagnosis and treatment fall far short of the remedial psychological treatment her condition demanded.

A fuller examination of the current wave of self-destructive activities suggests that self-inflicted injury is a small part of a larger scenario of hostile acts played out in our youth subculture.

Skin Wars

Psychiatrists appear to have missed the most dramatic statement of our youth: The skin is the new battleground for defining the self. As measured by the proliferation of clubs in major cities like New York and San Francisco where members intentionally engage in blood acts and skin cutting, an unknown but substantial number of adolescents and young adults currently engage in self-mutilation. Such mutilation was once grouped with attempted suicide as a call for help. But according to the participants, ritual piercing and "mutilation" is much more an act of affirmation, a declaration of uniqueness, and a rebellion against conformity. Clearly more is at stake than simple self-hate.

The New Iconography

The current American craze of deforming the skin through tattooing, piercing, and cutting is clearly a manifestation of something deeper than a subcultural fad. The popularity and intensity of skin games put skin mutilation at the apex of recent moves in the youthful cult of rave parties and heavy "indie" (independent) and hard rock music to intensify experience and sensation.

Today the flagellation that passed for veneration of the deity in previous centuries has been replaced by this new subculture of self-mutilation. As before, the focal point for these rituals of abuse is the skin. A recent issue of *Spin* magazine documents the extent of this obsession.[7] Although no formal surveys exist, skin mutilation is common among the survivors of abuse, as well as among prison gang members and gay and lesbian teenagers generally. The form taken by skin mutilation in this subculture goes beyond simple tattooing. In a perversion of the traditional ends of plastic surgery, skin mutilation has progressed to the use of scalpels, razors, scissors, Swiss Army knives, and even the surgical tools of the cosmetic surgery trade itself.

According to one observer, young people "cut" to get attention and even to *avoid* suicide by substituting controlled physical pain for an uncontrollable "nebulous inner pain."[8] The mutilation and quasi torture enacted at the body's surface in the youthful underground can be extreme: Intentional scars are created by repeated cuts and red-hot branding irons made of sheet steel. Students may be suspended from flesh hooks. Others are skewered with stainless-steel nails or rings or even nailed to a cross.

A typical acolyte has numerous tattoos; pierced ears, tongue, lips, navel, and/or nipples; and a body covered by a mélange of faint scars (called "hamburger cuts" in the trade) or more visible keloids. These latter skin scars are created by rubbing sage or other irritants into a wound to create a thickened, raised scar. Unlike tattooing, scarring has a vague semblance of an art form, but its significance appears more religious than artistic. Scarring appears to be a way of reclaiming one's own body and of making a statement of identity.

As in the mutilations of past religious cults like the Lakota Sioux practitioners of the Native American sun dance, where skin piercing was part of a rite of passage, the infliction of personal pain through the skin is also a sign of willingness to subordinate one's self to a higher force or another being. Today, the "other" may be a lover or dominant partner in a sado-masochistic act.

As suggested by the current spate of sex parlors that offer mutilation, sensuality and the skin are inextricably tied. Scarring in particular carries sexual overtones, and the resulting pain can promote a previously unattainable intimacy with a lover/abuser. One heavily scarred woman displaying a spiral of petal-shaped keloids right over her sternum described the cutting that produced it as a "psychic orgasm." The very intensity of the pain needed to make such scars often make them emotional centers of a person's existence, providing meaning where none existed.

The historical recurrence of the theme of skin mutilation may be linked to a deep-seated need to use pain to subordinate the self. The stigmata of Christ were once ritually self-inflicted on supplicants as a sign of devotion. Whatever the ultimate purpose of skin mutilation, some significant portion of modern youth appears to be resurrecting a primitive tradition, but without the pagan and religious trappings it once had.

The fact that the skin is the focus for this movement is no accident. It is the single most visible image we project to the outer world. When it is scarred or heavily tattooed, the skin may be a mute signal of inner wounds or a tortured self-image resulting from sexual abuse or other childhood traumas. Like the faint bloodstains on the Shroud of Turin that purportedly covered Christ's body, surface disfigurements may provide an outward sign of our innermost sufferings.

Pigment

Perhaps the most obvious psychological element of skin is its color. While this is not the place to discuss the cultural issues of racism, it is appropriate to remind the reader how deeply skin color is confounded with self-identity.

A wonderful case in point came about in the course of a genetic counseling session conducted in a Central Valley setting in California. In this situation, a Hispanic family was distressed about the social stigmatization they associated with the birth of their albino son. Although some forms of albinism are associated with blindness, this child could expect only a mild form of light sensitivity and little or no long-lasting retinal changes. In spite of this excellent prognosis, the father remained depressed about his son's stigma.

The counselor was able to bring out the fact that the father felt his child's condition reflected on his own manhood. When questioned closely about the reasons for his distress, the father explained that for the Latino culture, color was a sign of power and strength. He believed that his children were a signature of his manhood. Because he took responsibility for his son's condition, he felt ashamed by the boy's lack of color. Absent a ruddy complexion and a deep-toned skin, albino children were considered weak and impotent. After extensive counseling, the family was able to accept their newborn and even anticipate more healthy children, even though they carried a 25 percent chance of recurrence for this recessive form of the disease.

Elsewhere in the Caribbean, similar views prevail. In the Dominican Republic, people of color also stigmatize those who have albinism. In a predominantly mulatto community where the general population has a dark brown skin pigmentation, albinos are commonly stigmatized and set apart from the rest of the social group. Many feel a prejudice toward albinos that echoes that of the Mexican American family: albinism is associated with weakness.[9]

A similar judgment about skin color can be found in other communities. The American rock stars Johnny and Edgar Winter, both of whom suffer from a serious form of albinism, once described their own social ostracism in a largely rural, Appalachian community. In a recent interview, Johnny Winter recalled an acute awareness of his uniqueness, which led him to withdraw from his peers. In response, he invested heavily in a

kind of private meditation in his music. As he told his inter-
viewer, "You know the way kids naturally are if you're fat, crippled, or in any way defective. They tend to leave you out. So
music became my identity and replaced the normal activities
that otherwise would have filled my life."[10]

Ironically, the central myth about albinism's linkage with
weakness and impotence is turned on its head in other cultural
groups. A group of Nicaraguan Indians consider albinism to be
a sign of virility and sexual prowess. For Indian women, to have
sex with an albino man is considered akin to making love with
a god. For this reason albinism is highly prevalent within this
community, as many children are sired by the few albino males
around.

These anecdotal reports point up a central issue: What skin
color is favored by a particular group is determined more by
cultural idiosyncrasies than by any rule. However, one theme
that clearly runs across many cultures is a "natural" dominance
and higher social standing afforded to the lighter-skinned
members of a group with common cultural heritage.

In the 1950s and earlier, it was common for the American
Negro to aspire toward lighter-colored skin. Persons who used
skin lighteners or who were naturally light-skinned enough to
"pass for white" were afforded higher cultural status than were
dark-skinned African Americans. In India, the caste system is
even more formally stratified by skin color, with the highest
Brahmin class having the fairest and the Sudras or untouch-
ables having the darkest-pigmented skin.

The light-skinned Aryan peoples who dominated the Indian
subcontinent allegedly spread as far as Europe. In the Middle
Ages, the myth of Aryan superiority set in train a legacy of
racism that achieved its apotheosis in the Third Reich. Such
racism is seeing a resurgence among neo-Nazis both in Amer-
ica and in Europe. In Japan, those with near-white skin are also

given the highest status, as evinced by the color of the favored makeup of the geisha and kabuki player: pure white. And in China, fair-skinned northerners are afforded higher status than their darker, more southern counterparts.

All of this speaks to some common cultural selection that appears consistently to favor lighter-skinned individuals. One hint as to its psychocultural origins is in the roots of the penchant for light skin among Caucasian groups. In Appalachia, a folk tradition is that fair-skinned girls are considered more attractive than their darker-skinned peers. The difference relates to social class. As one writer described it, "My own grandmother, who grew up on a farm, abhorred sun-browned skin and used to scold my sisters and me to cover up, saying that we looked as if we'd been working in the fields all day. . . ."[11] The association of tanned, dark skin with lower-class, outdoor work is akin to the Chinese tradition of having royalty maintain impossibly long fingernails to signify that they never worked. A fair skin may thus have become a cross-cultural flag for upper-class status, as it implies a life of leisure protected from the sun.

Adaptation

We now know that pigmentation bears no relationship to biological fitness. If anything, darker skin is better adapted to environmental insults and solar exposure, having both less allergic reactivity (as measured in occupational contact dermatitis) and sunlight-produced damage. In the end, the type of skin that is afforded the highest social status is purely an acquired cultural feature driven by preference, style, and aesthetics. But it is the biology of the skin that determines its limits and ultimately defines our cultural predilections for changing it.

THREE

Anatomy Lessons

It is a common joke among dermatologists that no one dies of old skin. But if the skin if not a vital organ, it is certainly an essential one. Without it, we would die. If a substantial portion of our skin is damaged through trauma or a burn, the loss can be fatal. When the loss approaches 40 percent, it becomes difficult for the body to maintain fluid levels, and the kidneys are often stressed to their limits to keep a proper balance of salts in the blood. Even minor breaches in the skin's integrity can invite bacterial invasion, and serious losses can lead to fatal and intractable infections. The recent spate of deadly "flesh-eating" streptococcal bacteria that cost puppeteer Jim Hensen his life and killed several others throughout the country arose from bacterial invasion through otherwise minor skin scrapes or cuts. In one instance a Michigan man simply scraped a knee in a bicycle fall. Two days later he was dead. All of this suggests that the biology of the skin is more complex and important than may at first be appreciated.

In the past, anatomy texts described the parts of the skin as if they were static, independent appendages, akin to layers in a cake. But the skin's anatomy is a fascinating mélange of cells in constant flux and interdependence. The typical square inch of body skin includes some 19 million cells, including an average of 625 sweat glands, 90 sebum or oil glands, 65 hair follicles, 19,000 sensory cells, and as much as 4 meters or about 12–13 feet of microscopic blood vessels. These cells and organs are integrated into the various structures that make up the skin as a whole.

Composition

🖎 Perhaps the cake analogy is understandable. After all, from birth on, the skin can be seen to be composed of three distinct layers. The thinnest layer is at the surface and contributes the cellular debris of dandruff and shed skin cells. It is called the stratum corneum or cornified layer and is typically about a tenth of a centimeter thick. Below it is the epidermis, consisting of five to thirteen layers of living cells and averaging about a half centimeter in thickness. Underneath the epidermis is the dermis, a layer averaging about 1.25 centimeters or just less than a half-inch thick, made up largely of collagen, fibroblast cells, and elastic fibers.

The Stratum Corneum

🖎 As unappetizing as it sounds, the most visible part of our skin's surface comprises sheets of keratin, the protein that gives the skin its internal strength, and the remains of dead, flattened cells called squames. This nonliving layer nonetheless plays a vital function as our basic barrier against dehydration. The uppermost portion of the stratum is normally moistened by contact with its underlayment of well-hydrated, viable tissue. But because of its proximity to the environment, it is vulnerable to drying out. Under adverse atmospheric conditions of wind, cold, and dry air, the stratum corneum can rapidly lose water and develop a firm and brittle surface.[1] As any ski and cold-weather enthusiast knows, should you persist in staying in a dry, cold environment, the skin will dehydrate. If left untreated, dry skin may crack, becoming painful and subject to infection.

Epidermis

Beneath the stratum corneum, the epidermal cells are divided into six discrete layers. Immediately below the cornified layer is a layer in which the lipids are produced that afford the skin its watertightness. When this synthesis is impaired, as occurs in certain genetic deficiencies (such as steroid sulfatase deficiency) or when drugs are used to reduce blood lipid levels, a chronically dry, scaly skin can result.

Below this layer are cells with a grainy appearance that make a protein called filaggrin, which in turn is assembled into keratin. Certain components of this keratin are made in the next layer of "prickle" cells, so named because of their sharp edges. At the very base of the epidermis are aptly named basal cells, from which all other epidermal cells are ultimately descended. Most of the pigmented cells of the skin, known as melanocytes, also reside near the base of the epidermis. Beneath all of these cells is a narrow, tough sheet of protein known as the basal membrane. The cells in the epidermis move constantly upward from their origins in the basal layer at this membranous interface to death at the surface.

Altogether this primordial skin cycle takes place over

twenty-eight days, from cellular birth to death. About half of this time is spent in moving from the basal layer into the stratum corneum. Cells that reach the stratum then flatten out, die, and are ultimately shed in the remaining two weeks. This seemingly insignificant observation has great significance to cosmetologists and anatomists alike, since almost any basic change in the composition of the skin will of necessity require three to four weeks, the time needed to move new epidermal cells to the skin's surface.

Dermis

Comprising primarily a tough elastic group of proteins called collagen and elastin, the dermis is a discrete layer underneath the epidermis. It is held in place by downward protruding pegs of skin known as the rete ridges, which normally keep the epidermis and dermis tightly wedded, much the same way the conelike outcroppings of a foam camping mattress prevent it from slipping on the ground. In a rare congenital disease where these pegs are lacking, the epidermis slips off its dermal bed and forms blisters or bullae that cause much discomfort and pain.

In the uppermost layer of the dermis, the connective tissue fibers of collagen line up vertically and form what is known as the papillary dermis. Below that is a group tightly interwoven with proteinaceous fibers, organized into a netlike reticular layer. This layer confers to the skin both elasticity and resistance to tearing.

The deepest dermal layer comprises fat cells interlaced with connective tissue. The thickness of these pads of fat gives the skin its characteristic contours, conferring thickness to the cheeks and minimal covering to the nasal cartilage. Anthropologists, knowing the typical thicknesses of this layer, can recreate a full face from a skull by adding layers of appropriately thick skin to the cheeks, jaws, and orbits. In some peoples, notably the Athapaskan Eskimo, this fat pad can be lifesaving. By affording wonderful insulation against the cold blasts of arctic winds, the padded cheeks of an Eskimo insulate the underlying sinuses and prevent the cold from penetrating to vital tissues. Elsewhere, notably at the mons venus, or Mound of Venus, dermal fat pads cushion the underlying tissue and bone and offer protection from impacts that might otherwise be bruising.

The miles of blood vessels that course deep within this dermal layer provide oxygenation and nutrients, and take away metabolic by-products and newly synthesized vitamin D precursors. Special cells in the dermis near these vessels known as mast cells (from the German for food or well fed) can release powerful substances under certain conditions that act on the blood vessels. Mast cell–released histamine causes profound blood vessel widening, or vasodilation—and in an allergic reaction known as anaphylaxis may produce so much vasodilation that the blood pressure plummets, leading to fainting, shock, and even death.

Deep within the dermis are smooth muscle cells that concentrate at special sites like the scrotum and nipples and around the hair follicles. Under sexual stimulation these muscle cells contract to cause erect nipples and retracted scrota and in the throes of a good childhood horror movie produce "goose bumps." Evolutionarily, the tenting effect of muscular contracture around a hair follicle probably arose as a mechanism to erect the hair in critical areas as a flight or fight response to threats and fear. The raised mane of a mastiff or guard dog, the erect hair on the arched back of a cat in a defensive posture, and the hair standing up on the back of your neck after a fright all have similar evolutionary roots.

Hypodermis

Some anatomists identify a fourth area beneath the dermis known as the hypodermis, which consists mainly of connective tissue and fat. It varies widely in thickness from 1.0 to 6.6 centimeters, depending on the nutritional status of its owner, because it is here that the most subcutaneous fat collects. In a picture of contradictions, the hypodermis is of paramount importance to two groups: Eskimos and body builders. As we have seen, because of added fat to this layer, Eskimos have a greatly increased tolerance to the arctic cold.

Body builders strive to reverse this process. A trip to any branch of Gold's Gym, where serious body building is under way, will almost always be rewarded with a discussion of how best to reduce this skin layer. When the competition season starts, body builders focus on stripping out the subcutaneous fat that otherwise hides the full definition of their muscles. Called "cutting," this process often involves strenuous dieting with additives like chromium picolinate and a process of intentional dehydration to minimize the amount of water retained in the hypodermis. Sometimes body builders will even use fat solvents in a misplaced effort to dissolve all remaining fat. A well-"cut" body builder will have less than 4 percent body fat, a level normally reached only among starvation victims or distance runners. The protective role of this layer is highlighted by the curious fact that in spite of their bulk, body builders who achieve the "cut" look are often cold all the time!

Life on Man

Our skin is host to a veritable entourage of microorganisms during its short life. As many as twenty million bacteria and fungi and numerous parasites and arthropods inhabit each square inch of our skin. We are not born so colonized, but rather acquire this ecological microcosm in stages. Prior to birth, the skin and its slippery, waxy secretion known as the vernix caseosa remain a sterile enclave. Beginning with delivery, as the baby passes through the vaginal canal, it picks up a number of indigenous bacteria and viruses. Should the mother be HIV positive, it is here that the infant is most likely infected.

After birth, the sterile skin is seeded constantly by individual bacteria and fungi, including various staphylococci, corynebacteria, streptococci, and occasional coliforms. These interlopers land on the skin much as invaders would colonize a vacant planet: tentatively and with many failures. But certain bacteria are "intended" to thrive on the skin and are remarkably successful in expanding from their initial landing sites rapidly.

Within the first day of life outside the womb, a baby's skin is almost entirely covered with a thin film of bacteria contributed by the mother. Most of this new flora is either beneficial or neutral in adaptive value. Some misguided efforts to sterilize the mother's skin may actually be counterproductive, since the infant commonly depends on the natural, bacteria-related scents that characterize its mother's unique odor to find the nipple. Conversely, nursery studies have shown that mothers can recognize their own babies by the particular odor they acquire from the bacterial hosts on their own skin.

The key study that proved that newborns also rely on skin

odor was performed at the Tatus Hospital in Estonia. A team of pediatricians found that washing one of the new mother's breasts and nipples led the infant to seek out the unwashed one for its first nursing. Within one to two hours of birth, twenty-two newborns found and nursed from their mothers' unwashed nipple, compared with only eight who chose the washed one.[2] Like many others, this study demonstrates the importance of retaining a healthy skin flora. In the face of hundreds of ads urging daily lathering, this goal may prove elusive.

Shortly after birth, in the warm, moist confines of the newborn's armpit, some 6,000 bacteria can be found on every square centimeter of skin. By day five, this density has increased to 24,000 per square centimeter, and by the ninth day postpartum, the bacterial population plateaus at about 81,000 on every square centimeter of skin.

One population of natural bacteria involved in this colonization is vital for the infant's well-being. In fact, they "belong" on the skin. When the mother first touches her new infant, she seeds it with her own skin bacteria, including some members of the genus *Bacillus*. At the breast, the infant's skin picks up the bifidus (or forklike) bacteria known as *Lactobacillus*. These same bacteria colonize the healthy infant's gut and are excreted by the billions in the fetal excreta.[3]

Should this natural chain of benevolent maternal contagion be broken, as can readily occur in premature and bottle-fed infants, catastrophe may lurk just around the corner. Should an infant who is unprotected by a natural coating of these lactobacilli be handled by a nurse carrying a pathogenic strain of staphylococcus bacteria, a serious infection can ensue. In one instance, a single staph carrier contaminated the skin of nine out of thirty-seven bottle-fed babies whom she had handled within their first twenty-four hours after birth. In another group of thirty-one who had also been handled by this nurse but who had ample contact with their mothers through nursing and fondling, no infants became ill.[4]

Later in life, the skin becomes colonized with other bacteria. Until puberty, these bacterial populations remain largely in check and in balance with each other. However, once the hormonal surges of puberty stimulate the sebaceous glands' secretions, all bets are off. Acne-accelerating propionibacterium (named after their ability to release propionic acid) proliferate in vast numbers. Before taking antibiotics or other medications in a well-meant attempt to destroy these bacteria entirely, one should remember that others are distinctly beneficial. As we saw with the breast-fed infants, these and other natural flora protect the skin and mucous membranes of the mouth and throat from their genuinely harmful counterparts like *Streptococcus pyogenes* and *Staphylococcus aureus*, both of which can readily colonize antibiotically disrupted skin. Other denizens of the skin, notably *Micrococcus luteus* and *Streptococcus mutans*, also afford direct protection against these more dangerous invaders. The range of disease-causing bacteria that the normal skin flora and fauna inhibit is remarkable and include pathogens that cause meningitis, intestinal inflammation, lung and throat infections, and old-fashioned boils.

The skin thus carries a veritable entourage of bacteria that we are consciously or unconsciously assaulting daily with antiseptic-containing soaps and creams, detergents and solvents. Some of the more robust members of the genus *Bacillus* actually make their own antibiotics! (The next time you pick up a tube of topical antibiotic, look at its ingredients and you will see bacitracin listed: it was originally isolated from one of these bacteria.) Unfortunately, only about one in five Americans still carry these valuable bacterial allies. The rest of us have succeeded in annihilating what may have been an essential protector against skin infections and may be at increased risk of dangerous staph and strep infections like the one that killed Jim Hensen.

The Nature of Skin

This ecological view of our most important organ must include another central feature: unlike any other organ except perhaps for the intestinal tract lining (our internal skin), the cellular populations of the skin are constantly being replenished. Every day, in addition to billions of dead skin cells, we shed an average of two hundred hairs. In turn, the skin replenishes these losses with more tissue and keratin. Should that cycle be interrupted by abrupt hormonal changes or chemotherapy for cancer, the skin may die a little. Hair falls out, the epidermis thins, and elastic fibers may be lost—and not replaced. In part, this process occurs as we age, but never so dramatically as when we are sick or chemically treated by radiation or agents that slow down or halt the replication cycle in the skin.

Some animals avoid the potentially catastrophic loss of their fur covering during starvation by committing only portions of their body surface to regeneration of hair at any one time. A "hair cycle" lasting from four to five days occurs splotchily over the bodies of rodents and other densely furred animals like chinchillas, much to the dismay of furriers who look for uniform pelts. When a field of skin cells is in an active phase of hair cycle, blood vessels become locally engorged and new keratin is produced vigorously in the hair follicle. This protein is shaped into the cylindrical hair shaft as it is extruded from the follicle at the skin surface.

In spite of the assertions of legal evidence technicians to the contrary, you cannot tell the genetic makeup from the "hair" of a person—it contains only dead keratin material. But at the base of any full-length piece of hair is a hair bulb or follicle in which a handful of cells will exist. In humans, only about fifty to one hundred follicles go into their active hair production cycle in any given day, and then only at random and not in the intense patches that characterize fur-bearing animals. After several years, an actively growing follicle stops and the keratin-producing skin cells around the hair shaft wither and withdraw downward, leaving only a tiny bulb of vital cells at the hair base. Hairs may be shed at this point, providing a source of cellular matter (if the hair bulb is intact) that can be used for DNA analysis and ultimately for fingering a suspected assailant or culprit. If shedding does not occur, the hair follicle may recover after a resting period of up to several months and commence making hair again.

Interconvertibility of Skin

As anyone with a mirror knows, hairy skin in one portion of the body can give way in another to a desert of naked or "glabrous" smooth tissue lacking hair altogether. Scar tissue may have no hair follicles or sweat glands at all. In many animals, the skin can also form a remarkably thick and robust pad of tissue at the bottoms of the paws. But most remarkable of all is that the epidermal cells taken from any of these areas can interconvert to the proper thickness, hairiness, and toughness characteristic of a new tissue site. This means that the thickened, highly specialized cells of the tongue could actually pave the soles of the feet and vice versa if experimentally moved there. Over the proper dermal pavement, epidermal cells will readily make new hair follicles.

The secret of this remarkable fact was discovered in 1967: the type of skin that forms on our body is directed by the underlying dermis. If placed over the dermis of a denuded footpad, suspensions of epidermal cells from any body location become footpadlike in thickness. Nearly hairless epidermis from the ear becomes hairy when transplanted to a haired location on the body proper. Even the normally hairy epidermis of the body will develop the characteristic papillae and taste buds of the tongue if placed on that organ.[5] Much to the dismay of early plastic surgeons (and their patients), the converse is also true. If skin grafts are made with the dermis intact, the skin will retain its characteristic hair pattern and direction. This means that if shaven "full-thickness" skin from the buttocks is placed on the face to cover a burn wound, the resulting skin will have the hair pattern of the site of origin. Only if pure epidermal cells are used and enough viable dermis remains at the site of injury will skin acquire a semblance of normalcy.

While this singular observation is almost thirty years old, the current generation of cosmeticians has apparently failed to grasp its importance. If the dermis is what determines the quality of tissue that grows above, the condition of the dermis determines the quantity and form of the resulting tissue. This means that if the dermal factors that make for the rich, thick epidermis of an infant's cheeks could be isolated and injected beneath the atrophying facial skin of an adult, regeneration to its childlike form would be possible.

Hairlessness

While the major features of the skin's anatomy have been amply described, its most obvious one remains a mystery: it's just so, well, naked! Anthropologists and evolutionary researchers alike have been stymied for centuries to explain why humans have so little hair on their bodies. How did this hairlessness evolve, and what possible function does it serve?

When it comes to hair among land mammals, we humans stand out almost alone. With the possible exception of the pig, nude mole rat, and the elephant, no animal is as profoundly naked and vulnerable as we are. We are indeed, as anthropologist Desmond Morris once said, "the naked ape." One clue is that human skin is unique for one other reason. It is shot through with sweat glands. One of the more common myths about skin is that this state of glabrousness, a more polite term anatomists use for nakedness, renders humans vulnerable to the elements.

No one who has shivered in a cold bathroom after taking a shower will deny a certain weakness of our anatomies for want of insulation. But humans have the ability to acquire a quite sufficient secondary defense against cold. Not unlike our nearest mammalian skin kin, the pig, humans have retained the capacity to lay down fat underneath the skin as a buffer against wintry blasts. As we all know too well, given the proper diet and a sufficient amount of time, it is all too easy to thicken our subcutaneous fat layer. This predilection to put on subcutaneous fat is both a boon and a bane. For Mongolian peoples living near the Arctic Circle, a one- to two-centimeter layer of fat is a marvelous adaptation against the cold, especially when it is laid down on the cheekbones. But for a person who has triggered this reaction as a result of overeating, excess fatty deposits can be distinctly maladaptive and can lead to years of often fruitless dieting and fasting.

No Sweat

But it is difficult to conceive of fatty skin as a raison d'être for hair loss. It is much more likely that the ability to acquire a thickened insulation of fat is a secondary adaptation necessitated by the loss of insulating hair. Answers to the skin's hairlessness may be closer to the surface. We may find clues if we examine the origins of the body's adaptations for releasing excess heat. Having a high density of sweat glands at the skin's surface provides a highly efficient mechanism for permitting the rapid cooling of the body's core through evaporative water loss—as long as this evaporation can proceed unimpeded by a hair coat. As might be expected, people who live in the tropics have higher densities of sweat glands in their skin than do those who have evolved in more temperate climes.

But evaporative cooling is a very expensive proposition from the body's perspective. Unlike panting, which uses the lungs to dissipate internal heat directly, sweating requires immense amounts of water. And in times of psychological stress, excess sweating appears distinctly maladaptive. It is neither a very adaptive response nor an effective means of reducing the "heat" of debate or argument. Nonetheless, sweating is an efficient cooling device in the tropics, where water is ample and evaporative breezes plentiful.

On a typical temperate day, the human body will sweat out about a liter of perspiration. Most of this is water, with a smattering of salts and waste products. On a hot day, the body will disgorge up to ten liters of sweat and often up to a liter per hour, fluid that must be replaced rather quickly or dehydration may set in.

If, as suspected, humans evolved in hot, lakeside environs where water was not a limiting factor, extreme glabrousness could have evolved in order to facilitate the cooling accomplished by sweat glands, leaving hair only on those surfaces that required protection from the sun (such as the head and, in males in particular, the arms and shoulders).

But the pattern of our hairy surfaces suggests another factor at work: sexual selection. The predilection of one or more of our ancestors for a particular distribution of hair readily explains the swath of genital and beard hair that make up our secondary sexual features. Sexual selection might account for loss of hair in males and its special distribution on secondary sites, but it hardly explains why females are even more hairless. Genital hair may have been sexually selected, but it also has a fundamental function as revealed by its resilient, kinky form: it buffers sensitive tissues against physical impact and abrasion during intercourse. But sexual selection alone would hardly explain the loss of a dense, hairy mat on virtually all of our remaining body surface.

Whatever its origins, the absence of hair links us most closely to a few diverse species like elephants and hippopotamuses. And here may be a significant clue: Both of these large mammals depend on water or mud for cooling themselves and for ridding their bodies of parasites and noisome insects. Could it be that we humans lost our hair in part as a defense against mites, lice, and fleas, which otherwise inhabit our more hairy counterparts, the chimps and apes?

No one who has seen gorillas or chimps at a zoo or seen movies of primates in the wild can fail to note how much time is spent in mutual grooming. Nor need we be reminded that

head and pubic lice, bedbugs, ticks, and other assorted parasites can still sometimes abound in the remaining hairy confines
of our own bodies. Each of these insect creatures has special
anatomical adaptations for holding on to hair. Loss of hair
would have denied the more threatening, disease-carrying versions of these arthropods a literal toehold, making their detection and removal infinitely easier. (Just consider how much more
difficult it is to remove a tick from the scalp than from an exposed area of skin.) Evolution would then favor the hairless versions of our ancestors, who were better protected from
anthropod-mediated diseases while allowing a residuum of this
dense scalp hair to remain for defensive purposes. Facial hair is
likely to have responded to sexual selection and served as a modicum of protection against injury to vulnerable areas on the neck
and face, where major blood vessels course close to the surface.

If hairlessness increased fitness in the face of arthropod-
borne disease, evolutionary processes must have led to other,
more subtle, social cuing and bonding mechanisms in primitive
human groups to replace the prior value of mutual grooming.
Social bonding habits, like group arrowhead making or weav-
ing and associated verbal communication, may have replaced
some of the social functions of mutual grooming and caused
further relaxation of natural selection for hairy humans. If this
is true, new social bonding, through vocalization and other
forms of touching, as well as the cultural drive to clothe the
body, may have evolved as a result of skin-related evolution.

Keeping Cool

🎐 But, you may ask, is not nakedness per se a liability? Not
in a hot climate. A naked skin cools the body far more efficiently than does a hairy one by allowing the rich interlacing

network of blood vessels that course through it to dissipate heat more efficiently. This efficiency derives from the extraordinarily rich blood supply that courses through the dermis just beneath the skin surface. Under normal conditions, an astonishing 3.3 percent of the heart's output of blood goes through the dermis, with another 2.2 percent going through the hypodermis. When the body's temperature rises, the blood vessels in both these areas dilate, permitting still more blood to go through the skin. So much blood goes through this system that abrupt dilation of these vessels can lower the blood pressure precipitously, leading to syncope or fainting. With the resulting movement of core blood to the surface, the body's blood supply is cooled down, just as hot water coming from your car's engine is cooled by coursing through the "vessels" of your car's radiator.

As we age, the blood vessels under the skin thin out and the resulting density of the capillaries running under the skin diminishes. The end result is a paling of the skin as blood tends to stay in the core of the body. This blood vessel loss may also explain why older people feel "cold." In fact, as gerontologist Leonard Hayflick points out, skin temperature—especially in the face—declines with age. The natural gradient of declining skin temperature from the body core to the extremities also is accentuated with aging. Cold feet is no myth. In some older women, the temperature differential from their groin to their feet can be as much as twenty-nine degrees Fahrenheit!

The elasticity of the blood vessels within the hypodermis also diminishes with age. In young people, these blood vessels undergo a rapid and predictable constriction after exposure to the cold, forcing more of the circulation into the body core. The resulting conservation of heat can be lifesaving should the skin be wet or the person immersed in cold water. Among the elderly, where skin blood vessel constriction is impaired, rapid loss of heat through the unprotected skin can produce a fatal case of hypothermia even under modest cold conditions.

Hairlessness Is Not Cool

While ample evidence exists to argue that hairless, sweat-gland-rich skin provides benefits in hot, dry climates, it is not the full story. The hairlessness is "cool" argument loses ground when we note that humans have selectively retained hair over precisely the exposed surface most in need of cooling, the head. The human scalp has about one hundred thousand hair follicles, slightly more in blondes, slightly less in redheads. Certainly the hair up there is not a universal adaptation, as male baldness is a commonly inherited condition (most often on the X chromosome) without major loss of life or limb. The scalp is richly crisscrossed with blood vessels but lacks sweat glands entirely. It is possible that in some cultural groups like the Masai or Bantu, who spend considerable periods exposed to the sun, the hair on the head serves as a secondary radiator of heat. But this explanation fails to account for the fact that many Africans, like the forest pygmies who have been confined to the shaded glades of the tropical rain forest for many centuries, if not millennia, have retained the same head of hair as did their more exposed savanna neighbors.

All of this reinforces the idea that some powerful selective force—like my proposed hypothesis of reduced risk of arthropod- or insect-borne disease—led to the abandonment of our hairy coats. Some such adaptive value must offset the obvious risks of hairlessness. There is a clear downside to emerging naked into the tropical sun. As virtually hairless mammals, we humans are in constant peril of sun-induced damage and dehydration. This state would seem to be more vulnerable than adaptive. How do we survive the risk of solar injury, overheating, and water loss?

For one thing, our unique upright posture greatly reduces the surface area exposed to the sun, leaving only the top of the head and shoulders exposed at midday. Also, the skin of humans is unique for its ability to darken after sun damage. And most of the peoples who inhabit the tropical regions of the planet have retained the initial melanotic pigments that shielded the skin and the rest of the body from the most harmful of the sun's rays. But solar damage, as we will see, remains a major concern for modern humans worldwide.

Even after all of this anatomical review, we are left with substantial uncertainty about the skin's basic purpose. Is it to serve as a heat exchanger and barrier against the elements, shielding us from sunlight and chemical intrusion; or may it actually be designed to permit access to the body, albeit a selective one, of certain vital radiation and nutrients?

FOUR

Form and Function

In spite of centuries of study, the full appreciation of just what the skin does has lagged behind the detailed description of its anatomy. Many of its key attributes have been fully appreciated only in the last two decades. Part of the explanation for this delay is the presumption that the skin is a passive covering—a flat, two-dimensional organ.

As our review of skin anatomy already shows, superficial appearances bely a tremendous amount of internal complexity. We have already recognized some of the functions of the skin. It provides us with "an edge" against a hostile environment, affording insulation, a heat exchange system, and a water-resistant cover. More critical functions like protection against bacterial and fungal invasion and a repair system to reverse the damage from ultraviolet radiation are just being appreciated.

Some elementary cues to these and other specialized activities are suggested by simple anatomical features. The calluses on our feet and the ridges on our fingers give their function away: they protect us from abrasion and increase the sensitive surface area of our fingers, respectively. Even seemingly minor perturbations in skin anatomy have great significance. The skin is exceptionally thin in certain areas like the scrotum and forehead, and in the region behind the ears and the inner or volar surface of the arm. This thinness makes the skin especially vulnerable to sensitizing chemicals and to permeation of substances that can diffuse through intact skin. Many potentially beneficial substances are able to penetrate the skin in these areas and to spread through the body because blood vessels are in proximity to the skin surface. As we will see in more detail in chapter 5, the skin's construction makes it selectively permeable to certain harmful chemicals.

In the last twenty years, drug companies have concentrated on these anatomical sites as ideal locations for the new class of drug delivery systems known as "dermal patches." Positioning a dermal patch over these skin "windows" permits the administration of drugs that need to diffuse continually into the body to assure their biological effect. At one time, drug manufacturers assumed that the skin route avoided metabolism of the drug because that route bypassed the liver's detoxifying system. But now, as we will see in more detail in chapter 7, the skin itself is recognized as having its own detoxification enzymes.

The thinness of the skin, especially in the scrotum, can be a bane as well as a boon. High permeability can put internal organs at risk for toxic injury. Should the folded, permeable skin around the testes be exposed to toxic chemicals, they may be absorbed. This has proven especially damaging in the case of spinning jenny operators and chimney sweeps. In these professions, testicular exposure to nitrosamines in cutting oils and benzoapyrene in soot has led respectively to testicular and skin cancer, a topic discussed at greater length in chapter 6.

Other modifications of the cutaneous layer have clear adaptive value. A semitransparent skin is essential for the proper functioning of the light-responsive pineal gland deep in the skull, which regulates our sleep-wakefulness cycle. And while thin, the eyelids and lashes provide a vital function in protecting the eyes against dust and dehydration. Special skin appendages like nails and hair once provided essential adaptations for defense.

Body Burden

For the skin to do all of these things means that the body has to maintain and repair it regularly. Given that the skin is the largest organ in the body, accommodating its metabolic demands for constant replenishment is no small matter. Restoring the billions of cells lost daily at the skin's surface requires a substantial protein and calorie investment by itself. In a 140-pound person, the skin weighs about twenty-two pounds, or about 16 percent of body weight, and accounts for about 5–8 percent of the body's metabolic demand. As we saw, the core of the skin's vitality lies deep within the dermis, where blood vessels provide a steady influx of nutrients. Under conditions of starvation, the skin can be seen to thin dramatically, making it vulnerable to infection and subject to greater heat loss. Winter deaths in Nazi concentration camps were often due as much to hypothermia secondary to starvation as they were to disease.

Healing and Renewal

As we saw in the previous chapter, skin cells progress through different stages of development until they slough off in a perpetual, silent shower of dead cells and debris. Some two to three billion cellular remnants are shed daily. Enough comes off the foot alone to add 190 mg of dead cells to a pair of socks. Each of us has a genetically unique scent coded in this discarded skin. At some primal level, it is this scent that attracts (or repels) our mates.

As shown by studies in the Pacific Northwest involving wet-suited adults "lost" in the woods, this constant rain of detritus provides the cues for following bloodhounds. When both suited and unsuited victims were tracked through the woods, only those whose skin was exposed were found. Without a skin trail to follow, hounds failed to track even a single rubber-suited victim. This fact is not lost on old "convict escape" moviemakers: having your prey dash through a stream breaks the trail of shed skin cells and throws off the bloodhounds.

This same process of shedding, or desquamation, that gives us all dandruff at some point in our lives is recognized by beauticians as the apotheosis of healthy, vibrant skin. Through a process of exfoliation, the accelerated stripping of soon-to-be-dead superficial epidermal cells provides an extra stimulus to the underlying basal layer to make new cells. The Japanese regularly rub the skin with rice to achieve this end, while cosmetic companies sell a whole range of products designed to gently abrade and desquamate the skin for the same purpose.

This capacity for renewal is what gives the skin its remarkable capacity for healing. After a wound, the underlying tissues form a blood-vessel-rich granulation layer over which epidermal cells migrate and proliferate. Intercellular hormones such as epidermal growth factor are released that push cells into faster division cycles, allowing replenishment of missing skin. Interestingly, the impetus for searching for this hormone came from observing animals that licked their wounds: epidermal growth factor was first isolated from the salivary glands. Today, new research indicates that this critical hormone is essential for the normal development of the skin and other epithelial structures like the lungs. In animals who lack a normal receptor that permits this factor to work in its target tissues, skin and hair fail to form normally and the lungs are underdeveloped.[1]

At the Surface

& If we were to single out the key role the skin plays, it would clearly be that of a protectant. The main function of the epidermis is to pave the body with an even, compact coat of tough protein. This keratin layer, which we described in the previous chapter, comprises a group of at least four related proteins from which hair and fingernails are also made. As cells move upward from the basal layer, they make more and more of this protein, until finally, at the uppermost layer at the very top of the stratum corneum, only keratin itself—and cellular debris—survive. The keratin layer is a tough, horny, and ultimately dead sheet of interwoven proteins.

As proof of its resilience, keratin (and not bone) is the principal component of rhinoceros horn. Because keratin is most commonly associated with hair, some anatomists once erroneously believed that this horn was just a compact hair mass. In fact, rhinoceros horn contains a highly compact and tough form of keratin as well as traces of luteotrophic hormone, a chemical that may account for the Asian belief in the horn's aphrodisiac power.

Ultimately, it is this compact layer of keratin that makes our bodies water-resistant and tough. These barrier functions of the skin depend on the initial synthesis of enough keratin layer at the skin's surface before the body is fully ready to interact with its environment. A fully protective keratin layer develops only in the weeks after birth. Before then, the fetus is covered with the already mentioned vernix caseosa, a cheeselike material of dead cells and waxy secretions. This slippery material is the bane of many a midwife and obstetrician and probably serves the infant as a lubricating barrier while in the womb that protects against abrasion. As proof of this protective function, very early premature infants (those born before twenty-eight weeks of gestation) who lack a keratin layer altogether are extraordinarily vulnerable to bruising and water loss. Such infants are commonly sheathed in Saran Wrap or other waterproof plastic to protect their delicate skin and to prevent dehydration.

One clue to the importance of this keratin is that some 95 percent of the cells of the skin are devoted to making it. The resulting keratins are assembled into a stiff, weblike pattern within the cell and form attachment sites at the cell borders that function like reinforcement bars in cement. This intracellular keratin thus confers physical strength to the epidermis as a whole. Some children are born with defects in this keratin layer. Six different genes are involved in making keratin, and when gene mutations occur in them, any of four distinct congenital defects can arise. As might be expected from its contribution to the skin's surface, some of these defects show up in the epidermis in the form of bullae or blisters. The location and severity of the resulting blistering depends on the cell layer in which the mutation produces a defective keratin.[2] Rarely, the keratin layer is thickened and unnaturally loose in a hereditary form of ichthyosis. The result is a thickened, "fishlike" scaly skin that puts its holder at risk of infection and desiccation. Another defect can lead to the overproduction of keratin or hyperkeratosis. Hyperkeratosis is also one of the features of psoriasis, a disease discussed at length in chapter 6.

Scarring

A common myth is that skin that is cut or torn will inevitably scar. Scar tissue itself is simply a massing of specialized cells known as fibroblasts where normal epidermis and dermis would be. The importance of minimizing scarring is both cosmetic and practical. For some individuals, excess scar tissue is a terrible problem. These people commonly form extra-dense growths of fibrous tissue known as keloids, and the simplest cut on the face or arms can be disfiguring. Scar tissue is also much more fragile than normal tissue. Lacking the normal abundance of elastic fibers and collagen, scars are prone to tearing and are a particular problem in gynecologic surgery where stretching and tension can pull at wound edges.

Until recently, the raison d'être of scarring and the means to minimize it have been poorly understood. The newest developments have been precipitated by research that has revealed the remarkable fact that the fetus generally forms no scar tissue at all after injury or incision.[3] Certain properties of young fibroblasts appear to help the fetus heal without forming a scar. Researchers who have examined this unique process have noted greatly reduced inflammation at the site of fetal injury compared with that of a newborn or adult. This key discovery hinges on the fact that the fetus generates very low levels of substances that excite inflammation (known as cytokines). In time, researchers may be able to inhibit the overproduction of certain cytokines and thereby minimize scarring in adults.

Skin Changes

*Most surgeons will wax prolific in describing the toughness of some of the human skin they have encountered, especially skin exposed to the elements. But there appears to be a biological basis for toughness that transcends experience. My own surgical experience in mice and rats provided a real eye-opener. Sex is the key determinant of skin resilience. In shaving a bed for a skin graft, I could cut through the thin layer of a female mouse's body skin with ease. But should I be unlucky enough to have to work with a male, I could barely cut the surface of its skin before my scissors would dull and my patience fray. This was especially true if the male were a fighter, since wounded skin was even tougher, stiffer, and more uneven than the untrammeled skin of a young adolescent male.

Besides basic biology that makes males "tougher" than females, a second lesson is that skin changes. In youth, it is naturally supple and mobile. Under the stress of physical abuse, it toughens appreciably, sometimes almost overnight. An abraded foot will deposit extra layers of keratin to make a callous in a remarkably short period—although for most of us a blister or two will precede this adaptive response.

Even the otherwise fragile-appearing skin of a child is immensely strong. To tear it requires over twenty-five pounds of force applied laterally. With age, the tensile or tear strength of the skin itself, and of the scar line of healed wounds in particular, declines dramatically. And skin will stretch to extraordinary lengths, as anyone who has gone through nine months of gestation will attest. This radical ability to expand and increase in surface area if subjected to steady and slow pressure led to one of the most amazing inventions in plastic surgery in recent years: the skin expander.

Called the Becker Expander after its inventor, Dr. Hilton Becker, it is essentially a surgically implantable, inflatable saline balloon encased inside a silicone gel bag. The inner cavity of this device can be gradually inflated with saline through a tube and special connecting valve port accessible by needle just under the skin. This process takes place over a period of weeks, not exceeding six months, and can lead to an expansion of the outer diameter of the bag up to 1½ times its original volume. If blown up gradually in this way, the expander will stretch the skin to three or four times its original size in a matter of months, creating a pocket into which a molded piece of artificial tissue or a prosthesis may be placed. This surgical feat is often a psychological lifesaver for a woman who has undergone radical mastectomy and lacks sufficient skin to permit reconstructive surgery. With the Becker Expander, she can often be outfitted with a breast prosthesis just two to three months postsurgery.

The key to the success of the tissue expander is the sensitive response of the skin to changes in external tension. This stretching ability is achieved not so much by cell stretching as by *new* cells that divide and migrate to fill microscopic gaps as skin contacts are put under tension. As pressure receptors pick up the stretching produced by a slowly filling expander, the basal layer of the skin is induced to produce more cells. The intrinsic elasticity of the skin plus this proliferative response is what permits it to expand and mold to the increased size of the underlying tissue in pregnancy or to the expander in reconstruction surgery. To appreciate this critical attribute of the skin, one need only consider what happens when it is lost. In one disease state, skin elasticity is lost almost entirely.

A Case Study: Scleroderma

In ancient Greece there was a well-known myth of the snake-haired goddess Medusa, who had the ability to turn to stone all who looked on her horrendous visage. It is likely that the basis for this myth was the rare observation of individuals with a skin disease known as scleroderma, from the Latin for "hard skin"; it affects some nineteen out of every million adults. Until Perseus came up with the idea of turning his highly polished shield into a mirror to view this evildoer, Medusa succeeded in condemning dozens of would-be vanquishers into silent totems of failure. In a quirk of fate, it was one of the drops of blood shed by Medusa under Perseus' sword that were used by Athena to begin the cult of Asclepius, the basis for modern medicine.

In scleroderma, the skin loses its elasticity and gradually tightens around the body and especially the extremities, enveloping its victim in a deadly embrace. The scleroderma patient is typically a young woman aged twenty to forty-five. Most are described as "hidebound," lacking any skin movement at all over their underlying tissues. The affected skin contracts around fingers, hands, and feet alike, causing painful contractures that pull them into clawlike contortions. The skin around the mouth also constricts, until it becomes almost impossible for the patient to open her mouth to take food.

In some patients, the scleroderma remains localized in a form known as morphea, for the deadened sensation of the affected tissue. However, other forms are more insidious, and in time, the internal organs may be affected. One extreme form of scleroderma, known as progressive systemic sclerosis, is usually fatal, as vital internal organs become replaced with scar tissue.

Scleroderma commonly begins innocuously enough. The future victim experiences a strange blanching of the fingertips, often brought on by cold. The blanching is the result of blood vessel contracture and is typically followed by a rebound effect that leaves the digits red and swollen. This condition, known as Raynaud's phenomenon (after French physician Maurice Raynaud, who described it in 1862), is found in some 3–4 percent of the population at one time or another. Only a small fraction of those with Raynaud's go on to develop a full-blown case of scleroderma. Subtle skin changes, including pitting or ulcerations in the fingertips and characteristic changes in the capillary bed under the fingernails, signal the likelihood that Raynaud's will progress to full-blown scleroderma.

The disease itself is a consequence of a strange and troubling biological phenomenon. Under as yet unknown conditions, the body's immune system will turn on itself, attacking the body's own tissues in a perversion of the normal role of the defense system. In the case of scleroderma, the target appears to be collagen of a special type (type IV). Proponents of one model for scleroderma posit that collagen may be deformed by interacting with other substances. The resulting structural change makes the collagen "foreign" to the body, which calls in the "friendly fire" of the immune system to attack itself. The resulting immune attack appears to further cripple the collagen, distorting its normal structure and destroying its normal elasticity. Autoantibodies that signal this immune attack also arise, including some directed against other skin proteins like laminin, while others attack cellular components and enzymes. The end result of this concerted onslaught is to produce what textbooks describe as "an exuberant fibrotic reaction" made up of excess collagen and altered forms of other skin proteins.[4]

Among the many agents that are known to trigger scleroderma are silica dust, vinyl chloride, the solvent known as trichloroethylene, certain anticancer agents, industrially contaminated cooking oil, chronic vibration, benzene, the chemical intermediary known as phenylenediamine, certain epoxy resins, carbidopa, some contaminants of fermentation-produced hydroxytryptophan, and, possibly, silicone gel from breast implants.[5]

This diverse list is at first bewildering, since the existence of such a wide variety of precipitating agents would appear to confound any causal analysis. Yet a closer examination may be revealing. Many of the substances like benzene, vinyl chloride, trichloroethylene, and the phenylenediamines have the capacity to permeate the skin. Also, silica is a component of breast implants, and both they and the silicone formulated as silicone gel are known immune adjuvants. Toxic oil that resulted from industrial contamination of cooking oil in Spain in the 1980s and hydroxytryptophan, a contaminant of some preparations of fermentation of the amino acid L-tryptophan, both contain strong oxidants that can alter skin proteins. Finally, anticancer drugs are also known to be mutagens that can result in altered antigens capable of provoking an autoimmune attack.

All of these agents apparently work on a common mechanism in the body itself that permits it to engage in autoimmune attacks when activated inappropriately. Such a response challenges the evolutionary biologist to question why and how such a mechanism evolved. Is it possible that an autoimmune response that tightens and thickens the skin once had an adaptive purpose? Or is it simply a case of a misdirected process that evolved for other reasons, such as control of parasitic diseases of the skin? Whatever the explanation, the pathogenesis of scleroderma points out the continuing vulnerability of the skin to disruption and failure should the body's basic defenses be deranged.

Nerves

🖎 Skin also must permit our sensory contacts with the outside world to be meaningful. In the somewhat stilted language of a standard text of dermatology, "[S]ensory nerve endings that terminate at the junction of the epidermis and dermis carry important information to the brain regarding our external environment."[6] When localized morphea occurs in scleroderma, serious damage from burns and cuts commonly result. We rely on our sensations to feel a burning hot plate, as well as a silky smooth cheek or a frigid splash of water.

In all mammals, the nerves in the skin are of at least four different kinds. Just under the epidermis, nerves that end in Meissner's corpuscles are responsible for sensations of itching and light touch. Deeper within the dermis are insulated fibers that innervate the Pacinian corpuscles. These onion-layered miniorgans allow perception of pressure. Ruffini's corpuscles deeper in the dermis respond to heat in one temperature range, while Krause's end-bulbs pick up temperature changes at another.

Uninsulated nerves that terminate right at the dermal-epidermal junction are largely the ones responsible for detecting subtle pressure changes at the skin's surface. The deeper nerves, well insulated with myelin, have more weighty functions, including the perception of pressure, deep pain, and temperature changes. In aggregate, it is these nerves that give us our outer sense of self—and provide sensations of impending forces that may injure us severely. A wholly different set of nerve fibers constitute the motor nerves that regulate blood vessel thickness (and hence blood flow), the activity of the sweat glands, and the contraction of muscles.

In some areas of the hands, notably in the fingertips, the den-

sity of nerve endings can be more than 1,300 per square inch.
But this density does not measure up to the sensitivity reached
by other animals. Aided by highly innervated whiskers, many
mammals from moles to cats can distinguish subtle vibrations
in their environment by touch alone.

While our nerve endings may be somewhat less than the
norm in some cross-species comparisons, we are nonetheless
usually "in touch" with our environment, except in circumstances that put us at grave risk. Loss of skin sensation entirely
can be disastrous. Leprosy patients often lose skin innervation
in their extremities. As their disease progresses, they develop
clubbed or missing fingers. The layperson may improperly con-
clude that such losses are the result of denervation or perhaps
the mycobacterium that causes the disease. But the amputation
of fingertips and ultimately whole digits results only indirectly
from the loss of nerve endings destroyed by the lepromatous
bacterium. Lepers will commonly burn or lose fingers to injury
because no warning pain will be given and other sensations of
severe injury, such as smell, will go unnoticed until too late.

The resulting deformities of the extremities and the mistaken belief in the contagiousness of the disease has led to
much unnecessary suffering for leprosy patients. Islands like
Molokai in Hawaii were set aside as leprosariums. "To be
treated like a leper" is still common parlance and refers to the
medieval practice of banishing lepers to the countryside. Japan
still retains outdated laws enacted at the turn of the century
that condemn lepers to a life of social ostracism.[7] In each instance, the stigma that originally defined a leper was the loss of
fingertips or digits. Such tragic consequences are mute evidence of the importance of skin innervation.

Skin and Bones

In addition to its protective role, the skin must also be able to permit light to penetrate deep into the body. For there to be adequate calcification of the bony parts of the growing body, the skin has to allow passage of enough light to permit the body to synthesize vitamin D. As every schoolchild knows, sunlight is needed to make vitamin D. This is almost, but not quite, right. Contrary to popular belief, the skin does not synthesize this vitamin per se but instead makes its precursor, a molecule known as vitamin D_3. Its conversion product, vitamin D itself, regulates the deposition of calcium and phosphate in the bones. Vitamin D is not an essential vitamin except under conditions of reduced ambient light that prevent the synthesis of adequate amounts of vitamin D_3. Normally, only a tiny amount of sunlight is needed for the protection of physiological amounts of vitamin D. Even exposing a newborn's cheek to full winter sunlight for half an hour each day is sufficient for its vitamin D needs.

But in northern latitudes, where heavy clothing is the rule and sunlight is of short duration and low intensity for a significant part of the year, even this amount of sunlight may be lacking. Until recently, many countries where vitamin D supplements were not routinely added to milk still recorded episodes of rickets. The characteristic bowed legs of rickets results from incomplete calcification in growing bone because of a vitamin D–mediated deficiency in the calcium-depositing hormone known as calcitonin. When calcitonin is deficient during development, blood levels of calcium and phosphate fall below the optimum levels needed for bone mineralization.

Rickets was especially prevalent in nineteenth-century London, where industrial development produced a heavy, sun-occluding smog most of the year, or in dark-skinned persons living in northern climes, where skin pigmentation limits light penetration. In the 1920s and 1930s, rickets proved to be a particularly vexing problem among African Americans who lived in Montreal. Until vitamin D supplements in milk were introduced in the 1940s, lack of sunlight continued to be responsible for vitamin D–deficiency states in many people living in the northern latitudes. Rickets and its accompanying bone loss (osteomalacia) still occurs sporadically in Great Britain and the Scandinavian countries. Paradoxically, it also occurs—especially among young women—in the Middle East and India, where customs dictate that the body be virtually completely covered and exposure to the sun is reduced accordingly.

While many Americans now recognize bone calcium loss as a factor of aging, few realize that the skin plays an integral role in this process. As persons age, they tend to spend less time in the sun and secrete lower amounts of sex hormones and calcitriol, the critical precursor hormone that controls calcium metabolism. When both of these events happen, less vitamin D is produced, leading to lower deposition rates of calcium in the bones, and calcium absorption by the small intestine decreases.[8] The result is that bone loss accelerates rapidly both as sunlight exposure wanes and as the skin's vitamin D–synthesizing ability declines with age.

Letting Light In

As we mentioned in the discussion of anatomy, light must be allowed to penetrate deep into the skull to trigger the release of critical phasic hormones that control our sleep cycle and our seasonal adjustments to metabolic and other needs. Deep within the skull, the pineal gland (the primordial "third eye") serves as a light receptor to control these cycles. Like the retina, the pineal too has light-receptive cells, at one time a perplexing anomaly to anatomists who mistakenly believed its central location in the skull made light penetration impossible.

For this to happen, the skin must let some light through, but not too much. The American Indian people, like all those of Asian ancestry, have adapted to the need for modulating light penetration by developing a particularly thick keratin layer at the skin's surface, while most African peoples have extra amounts of melanin for the same purpose. If too much sunlight penetrates the skin, unhealthy levels of calcium may build up in the blood (hypercalcemia), leading to kidney stones and bony spurs.

The trade-off between some light, but not so much that the skin overproduces calcium-stimulating hormones, has meant that fair-skinned people are at risk for other light-induced damage, including accelerated aging and cancer. While the skin of blacks is remarkable for its resiliency and smoothness well into old age, it is no secret that white skin typically ages more rapidly, crinkling with crow's-feet and developing extensive creases and lines that form the basis for the multibillion-dollar cosmetic industry.

But in addition to permeability to light, the skin has a previously unrecognized ability to selectively let in other substances, the topic of the next chapter.

FIVE

Barrier or Sieve?

The anatomy that we see when we look at our own skin has evolved over the millennia that life has existed on earth. To appreciate and understand the basic functions that our skin serves, we need to look at its origins. What skin can and does do for us, and the potential pitfalls of our crude attempts to manipulate it, are best understood in an evolutionary perspective.

Origins

In the ocean where life evolved, cell walls—the predecessors of our own outer integument—were initially an unnecessary physiologic luxury. The conditions that spawned life remained compatible with the cellular fluid for untold millions of years. A simple membrane probably sufficed to hold in living stuff and exclude the nonliving. Even today, some lower life-forms among the bacteria (such as the so-called pleuropneumonialike organisms) do just fine without a cell wall at all. And the ability of penicillin-based antibiotics to block cell wall production has not deterred the survival of some targeted organisms known as L-forms that manage to persist without their outer coats even after an antibiotic attack.

While in the water, most primitive cells, and even the earliest multicellular animals, such as the tentacle-waving hydra we all studied in biology, lacked a rigid cellular exterior. Instead, their bodies were covered in two-celled membranes that were generally permeable to the elements without and within.

A "skin" or cell wall became a biological necessity when the environmental conditions that had spawned the earliest forms of life began to change. Once evaporation made the primordial seas saltier than the life in it, some form of barrier was needed for protection. As compared with living cells, oceanic salt water created an "osmotic gradient" that would otherwise force the original life-forms to give up water to their surroundings. As the dissolved solids in the oceans became even more concentrated, single cells that did not isolate themselves from a now hostile osmotic environment literally dried out, losing fresh water to their saltier surroundings.

Those with an early form of skin around their cells protected themselves from desiccation and collapse by actively excluding salts. Later, when fresh-water organisms evolved, a skin served the reverse purpose, shielding the organism from swelling from the influx of too much fresh water. Over time, multicellular organisms were under tremendous selective pressures to build this cellular skin into an osmotic barrier that would maintain the internal milieu of their bodies against any changes in the saltiness of their environment. This was accomplished partly by having the skin serve as a selectively permeable membrane that permitted dissolved salts to be excreted and fresh water selectively taken in. When the skin itself no longer served as a sufficient osmotic pump, a specialized organ evolved to accomplish the same thing. Recognizable today as the forerunner of the kidney, this primitive filtration system used a network of vessels arrayed in a countercurrent net or *rete mirable* to flush out excess salts and by-products like urea.

As the great anatomist Alfred Roemer observed, all fish carried this organ within, as a preadaptation for their transition to life on land. No matter how humid and dank the imagined primordial forests, once on land, animals needed to protect themselves from drying out. Most had to achieve this environmental protection while permitting flexibility and sensibility. For many phyla, it simply did not work to be locked into a casing that sealed off all contact with the surroundings. The organism had to have sufficient latitude in movement to permit it to eat, explore, and find mates.

Animal Skin

When the first amphibianlike creatures emerged from the ocean, their skin was barely able to provide a barrier to dehydration. In fact, with a few exceptions such as highly insulated desert toads, all amphibia to this day reproduce in a watery environment and must maintain a moist skin surface to survive. Some frogs have skin so thin and permeable that they can literally breathe through it, barely relying on their lungs at all. In the highly oxygenated water of fast-running mountain streams, certain salamanders all but guarantee survival by breathing through their hyperthin, oxygen-permeable skin, dispensing entirely with external gills.

As amphibians evolved toward a more reptilian form, the skin and eggshells thickened dramatically to provide a barrier against desiccation. Hardy reptiles today can survive in the

Gobi and Mojavi Deserts with barely any water loss because of their tough and water-impermeable egg casings and waxy, highly water-retaining skins. Mammals evolved from these reptilian ancestors, keeping a dry skin and solving the problem of dehydration during external development by allowing gestation to occur internally.

The present form taken by our human skin is thus a result of millions of years and dozens of evolutionary experiments with this common motif. While other phyla like the Insecta successfully fused an external skeleton with mobility by segmenting their development, the lineages that led to humans retained a more plastic and mobile external raiment. This new skin had to serve as an external protection in lieu of scales or plates, yet be flexible to permit rapid movement. The resulting skin thus achieved a compromise between rigidity and flexibility, permeability and watertightness.

Mammalian skin strikes a balance between the extremes of reptilian watertightness and amphibian water-permeability. As a reminder of our evolutionary origins, the skin still serves as a gas-exchange organ and a nutrient-absorbing membrane early in embryogenesis. Derived from the outermost layer of the embryo, known as the ectoderm, almost all skin is descended from cells that had their origins at the surface of the embryo.

The earliest embryonic form is called a blastocyst, a ball of cells that receives all of its nutriment from being bathed in serum and the uterine secretions. To survive, the preembryo required a highly permeable skin. Not until blood vessels formed to supply internal structures did the external membrane of the embryo lose its almost total permeability. The need for secondary, keratin-mediated protection against dehydration does not appear until after birth. By then we are clothed in an unusual membrane—a virtually hairless, three-layered organ that at the same time protects us from the more noxious elements in our environment yet continues to allow in certain external agents and chemicals. The resulting fabric that clothes us thus retains many of the properties of its original form, particularly those that derived from cells that were originally highly permeable to many different chemicals and gases in solution.

While this fact formed a cornerstone of nineteenth-century embryologic study, it was mysteriously lost on the earliest human anatomists who believed the skin to be impermeable. Ironically, the "discovery" that our skin is readily penetrated by many chemicals was an enormous and disturbing surprise to the scientific community.

Keeping Things Out

Today we know the skin as a kind of schizophrenic organ, both denying access to the body of some things and actively encouraging the passage of others. Through the middle of this century, the skin was seen predominantly in its barrier role, preventing water loss, keeping the body out of contact with most noxious chemicals, and inhibiting the ingress of bacteria through its "acid mantle."[1] Modern researchers, especially in the new field of occupational dermatology, now know too well that the skin is a much more subtle "barrier" than these attributions suggest. Under some conditions it lets water out, permits toxic chemicals in, and allows bacteria to reside within its own confines. Ironically, as we will see, the same construction of lipids and proteins needed to make the skin resistant to water makes it exquisitely vulnerable to the entry of certain undesirable chemicals that dissolve in lipids and proteins.

Delayed Appreciation

If the skin's vulnerable composition was known early in this century, how did the outdated view of the skin as an absolute barrier against a hostile environment persist so long? Part of the answer involves our worldview of the skin as an extension of ourselves, as entities separate from nature. Until recently, we have tended to think of the skin as our boundary, a watertight covering that enfolds ourselves and our organs and keeps them separate from the world out there. We visualize the skin in purely Euclidian terms, as a two-dimensional sheet that envelops us in a kind of perpetual Saran Wrap. Since the environment is perceived as inimical, the primary function of the skin must be to keep things out, as a shield against the elements.

In actuality, as we have seen the skin is a highly convoluted, vulnerable, three-dimensional landscape. The skin's anatomy is planar only at the physical level of its gross anatomy: it does have a continuous surface and carries a contiguous keratin layer at its outermost boundary. But the skin itself has valleys, ridges, and folds, much as does the earth's surface. And, like the earth, it is shot through with pores, holes, and channels that greatly increase its surface area and make it anything but a smooth, two-dimensional surface.

These interstices and pores are guarded by special water-resistant molecules, but some chemicals, especially those that dissolve lipids, can readily penetrate these openings. And organs like the sweat glands that let water out can also allow water and any dissolved contaminants in. Under certain conditions, the pores can admit dissolved gases and various fluids as well as bacteria and other microscopic invaders.

Water Resistance

🖐 As an owner of many a water-resistant watch, I can attest to the fact that "water-resistant" and "waterproof" mean two different things. My water-resistant watch sooner or later permits water to enter its casing, while my son's more expensive waterproof watch takes long-term immersion without leaking. The skin is much more like my watch than my son's.

Under most circumstances, the skin provides the body with a semblance of water resistance, just like my watch. When I'm in a shower, my watch *and* my skin do just fine. But in a hot tub, both suffer. The watch gets water condensation under its crystal, and my skin wrinkles up. Both are the result of water being taken inside the outer structure.

What distinguishes the skin from all other membranes is the same thing that distinguishes my watch from my son's: its fine structure and inner workings. The skin is actually designed to permit a constant flow of "insensible" water percolating upward from its deeper layers. Water penetrates the skin's surface in a slow ebb from the highly hydrated layers below. And while an oily surface layer normally retains most of this water and resists entrance of additional water most of the time, waterlogging will occur, especially after long immersion in soapy water that breaks up the oil barrier. You also know that the skin's barrier to water loss is imperfect if you have traveled for any length of time in the bone-dry air of an airplane cabin.

This water resistance but not waterproofness of the skin is due to the coexistence of two different pathways through its outermost layers. These pathways take the form of molecular sieves that interpenetrate the skin much as wormholes pass through ancient wood. In the skin, these holes are submicroscopic passages that are actually molecular tubes lined with either water-repellent (hydrophobic) or water-attracting (hydrophilic) molecules. The skin's lipid or fatty elements make up the hydrophobic channels, while special water-attracting molecules largely make up the hydrophilic ones. These channels are positioned underneath the skin like the honeycomb of a beehive. This structure provides tiny interstices where very small amounts of water can move from below the skin to its surface while presenting a large number of water-repelling molecules to the outside.

Such an arrangement permits the skin to be flexible and largely watertight (from the outside in), while permitting a controlled amount of water to seep constantly through the lower skin layers to the skin surface. In most circumstances, this salubrious combination protects and nurtures the skin's outermost layers and gives healthy skin its "moist, fresh look."[2] But this same compromise means that the skin is susceptible to the inward passage of certain environmental chemicals that can dissolve these lipid layers. This important new discovery is called "permeation." It is what permits the newest drugs to be put into your body through the skin on special patches and certain highly toxic chemicals to pass through your intact skin without your awareness.

Myths of Impermeability

The recognition of unintended permeation of chemicals through the skin is a recent and major scientific event. Permeability was largely unappreciated, even among the foremost dermatologists. As recently as 1957, Dr. Stephen Rothman, keynote speaker at the Eleventh International Congress of Dermatology held in Sweden, assured his audience that the skin serves as a waterproof and impermeable boundary to the outside world.[3] Within a decade, we learned that Rothman was wrong, seriously wrong, and that his view—shared by many dermatologists worldwide—has led to much unnecessary suffering. By 1968, we knew that many industrial chemicals, including some that can produce sterility or cancer, readily traverse this "impermeable" barrier.

Skin permeability has also led to the poisoning of many children and the elderly, especially after extensive topical treatment with pharmaceutical disinfectants or pesticides. Even healthy young adults have been poisoned by skin permeation of pesticides like lindane, commonly used to treat head lice.[4] Newborns have also been brain-damaged from treatments with hexachlorophene, a chlorinated soap, in misguided attempts to reduce their risk of bacterial contamination in a hospital nursery.[5] In each instance, the unsuspected route of poisoning has been the skin.

Ironically, the penetration of chemicals through the skin has been utilized by preliterate societies for millennia. Before the age of the hypodermic syringe, skin permeation was a favored method of drug administration for many cultures. The most ancient schools of medicine recommended the uses of skin poultices as a vehicle for drug delivery. Moxibustion, the ancient Chinese process by which herbs are ignited over acupuncture points on the body, is a well-known and standardized technique for accentuating acupuncture treatments, enhancing skin permeability, and administering medicine. Pleurisy and pneumonia were treated over thousands of years of history by putting poultices of balsamic and other irritants directly on the chest. In ancient Mesopotamia, drugs were commonly put on cloths or pieces of leather and strapped to the skin to encourage their entrance into the body.[6] And Native American practitioners routinely recognized the skin as a penetrable covering through which both poisons and medicines could be administered, especially if the skin was first heated to increase the underlying blood circulation.

Occupational Illness

In 1960, just three years after Rothman's misplaced emphasis, one of the classic cases of occupational poisoning was almost missed because of the failure to recognize skin permeation as the route of exposure. In Lathrop, California, at the Occidental Chemical Plant, which produced tons of a nematocide known as dibromochloropropane (DBCP), a mysterious episode occurred where first one and then a dozen workers found themselves unable to father children.

DBCP's development came at a time when California's agriculture was struggling with hordes of teeming wormlike creatures called nematodes that threatened the roots of a wide range of valuable crops, from grapes to almonds. Among a host of chemical alternatives, only DBCP had the capacity to sterilize its nematode targets once applied in the earth under vines and almond and fruit trees.

Some four years earlier, a researcher working for an industry producer of DBCP had found that the testes of male rabbits treated with this pesticide shrank dramatically after exposure. It was not until almost a decade later, after the human damage had occurred, that this startling but unreported finding came to light.

By the mid-1960s, rumors abounded in the men's locker room at Occidental. Among almost forty young men who worked with this potent chemical, not one had fathered a child. Occidental officials offered assurances that they had kept exposures to DBCP well within occupational limits. It was not until a television film crew came to record a day at the plant that the apparent became obvious: while airborne levels of the chemical might have been "safe," the repeated dipping and immersion of unprotected arms and hands in solutions of DBCP provided an ample opportunity for exposure. Indeed, later calculations showed that enough DBCP was being absorbed through the skin to account for the sterility of many of the workers. Under the hot and steamy conditions of the Occidental Chemical Plant, DBCP was going through the exposed skin of the workers like a knife through butter.

This experience underscored the vulnerability of workers to occupational exposure from skin contact generally and with this potent chemical sterilizant in particular. The California State Legislature was so incensed by these events that it authorized the state Department of Health to set up a unit especially designed to preemptively detect such hazards. In 1979 I was asked by Beverlee Myers, the head of California's Department of Health Services, to head up this unit. Known initially as the Hazard Alert System and later downgraded to the Hazard Evaluation System, my group was charged with identifying previously unrecognized chemical hazards in the workplace and providing a clearinghouse for toxicological data. In the course of working with this unit, I came across many other examples of chemical poisoning where the skin was the portal of entry. Several are excerpted here to provide a sense of the extent of "skin poisoning" as a previously underappreciated route of exposure to hazardous chemicals.

Case Studies in Skin Permeation

1. HERBICIDES

The unit's first case was that of William O. This forestry worker was part of a crew charged with the job of weed eradication in the Oregon redwoods. Because of a recent ban on aerial pesticide application, this crew had the job of hand-spraying herbicides like Tordon (a chemical that contained 2,4 dichlorophenoxyacetic acid salts). In the course of a day's work, William O. had become drenched with the spray and had accidentally sprayed himself in the face. He wore his wet clothing for the rest of the day until the crew returned to their campsite. There he changed clothes. Even though he felt "a little woozy," he continued working. The next day he reported to his supervisor that he felt as though he had "the flu," with body aches, a headache, and generalized fatigue.

Two weeks later, he noticed weakness in his upper body and developed an unsteady gait. He felt pins and needles in his arms and legs. All of these signs and symptoms are characteristic of what is known as delayed polyneuropathy. But where did it come from? A California Department of Food and Agriculture team of inspectors, headed by Dr. Peter Kurtz, diagnosed it as Guillain-Barré syndrome, an aftermath of a flu virus infection. Our team went up to Oregon, where William still was, and took blood and urine samples: he still had sufficient 2,4 D in his system to register positive.

One of my staff, Dr. Jon Rosenberg, who had investigated the pharmacology of 2,4 D, discovered cases where dermal exposure (such as where a gardener had been kneeling on a 2,4 D–soaked pad) had led to the same polyneuropathy experienced by William O. Based on our investigation and literature review, we issued a hazard alert concerning unsuspected skin absorption of this herbicide. Not coincidentally, our report was used by Vietnam War veterans who had also experienced polyneuropathy as an alleged result of Agent Orange exposure, since 2,4 D made up about half of the mixture used in this defoliant.

A second case involved even more toxic chemicals that were absorbed through the skin. The herbicide paraquat has been responsible for many deaths among agricultural workers, usually from lung fibrosis following airborne exposure. It is a widely used, potent herbicide administered to control weeds on crops and to destroy coca and marijuana plants. In the past, most of the serious injuries and deaths that we saw were among agricultural workers, including "flaggers," who marked the runs of airplane spray applications and inhaled the spray.

But in a report of two patients from France, *dermal* exposure appeared to be the predominant route. In 1994, a team of poison control experts described how one patient died from respiratory failure twenty-six days after deliberately applying the herbicide over his entire body in a mistaken belief that it would afford relief from scabies. The second patient was a pesticide operator who was repeatedly exposed from wet clothing to a much more dilute solution of sprayed paraquat. Most interestingly, he had a preexisting case of psoriasis, which probably increased the permeability of his skin to the chemical, since psoriatic plaques are extremely rich in blood vessels. He suffered lung and kidney damage but recovered over a period of several weeks.[7]

2. WOOD PRESERVATIVES

In 1980, I learned of a worker at a Sacramento, California, wood treatment plant who had developed liver poisoning. The product he was allegedly exposed to was a wood preservative known as pentachlorophenol, one of the most popular protectants in the lumber industry used against fungi and insect pests. When I examined his case, however, I was perplexed. The whole operation took place outdoors, or in winter, in an open shed. Ventilation was more than adequate to minimize the inhalation of fumes from the treatment vats. What, then, explained his poisoning? On further questioning, the young man revealed that he commonly dipped the wood pieces to be treated into pentachlorophenol vats with his hands gloved but his arms bare. Commonly, he would emerge with soaked arms, his shirt reeking of the chemical. Sometimes he would wear the damp shirt all day.

His illness was characterized by night sweats, unexplained raging fevers (hyperpyrexia), and weakness in his arms. His blood chemistry came back positive, not only for elevated liver enzymes that signaled damage to that organ, but for excessive levels of pentachlorophenol. He had been poisoned through his skin. But why weren't his co-workers, some of whom worked side by side with him, similarly affected? The answer gave the case an additional twist: He had a condition known as Gilbert's syndrome, a genetically determined condition affecting some 5 to 6 percent of the population in which the liver is weakened and hence vulnerable to this chemical attack.

It was not until 1987 that the consequences of dermal and inhalation exposure to pentachlorophenol were fully appreciated,[8] too late to help this worker and his colleagues. Today we know that sawmill operators and homeowners who live in log cabins or homes treated with interior pentachlorophenol-containing wood protectants are poisoned on a regular basis. Unless they take appropriate precautions against inhalation *and* dermal exposure, such as sealing in the product or, better still, buying a new home, they remain at risk indefinitely, as the product outgasses inexorably from unsealed, treated wood products.[9]

3. PESTICIDES

Pesticide poisoning from skin exposure is a hidden source of many farmworker illnesses both here and abroad. On the suspicion that highly suspicious symptoms were the result of a source of low-level, chronic exposure to organophosphate pesticides, a British team examined the neuropsychological performance of a group of 146 Australian sheep dippers.[10] Two or three times yearly, dippers run their sheep through a deep trough containing a concentrated pesticide solution to rid the animals of insect pests.

The dippers' exposure was almost entirely dermal, the result of being splashed, wearing pesticide-dampened clothing, and handling treated sheep. Compared with a group of 143 nonexposed quarry worker controls, the workers showed a dramatic and consistent impairment in their ability to pay attention and process information, subtle signs of organophosphate poisoning. Most interestingly, the dermally exposed sheep herders showed an increased predilection to psychiatric disorders, a phenomenon previously noted only among workers heavily exposed to organophosphate pesticides via the airborne route.

4. DISINFECTANTS

The skin also provides a clue to explain a previously unappreciated health risk. The risk results from absorbing chloroform when bathing in heavily chlorinated swimming pools. (Chloroform forms as a result of chlorination of water containing humic and fulvic acid or other organic matter.) A research team from Quebec assessed the amount of chloroform acquired from waterborne exposure by evaluating the exhaled air of swimmers after an hour in the water: the levels reached were significantly greater than any nonoccupational levels previously measured. From a starting average of 52.6 ppb the swimmers reached 1,093 ppb after their swimming workout.[11] (The high starting level is likely the result of breathing air in the pool environs already contaminated with chloroform.)

The portion of this exposure due to inhaled versus absorbed chloroform has not been determined. But it is clear that swimmers encounter substantial risks of chloroform poisoning from repeated and constant exposure to swimming pool water. Given the common use of bleaches and other disinfectants that contain or readily produce chloroform, a hidden risk of skin contact and absorption may also exist among householders.

5. BENZENE

Benzene is a universal contaminant of gasoline and is widely used in the manufacture of rubber. After an hour of exposure to benzene on an area of skin equal to both arms (approximately 100 square centimeters), an average worker will have absorbed 20–70 mg, a substantial dose of this carcinogenic chemical.[12] Researchers abroad have known since at least 1961 that workers in contact with benzene will absorb it through the skin,[13] but no governmental agency took action to limit this route of intoxication until almost thirty years later. As a result, service station operators and rubber industry workers have been at increased risk of at least one form of leukemia (acute myeloblastic leukemia) for at least three decades, even as new standards for protection against airborne benzene have lowered exposure from 100 to 1 ppm over an eight-hour workday. It was not until 1992 that the U.S. Environmental Protection Agency (EPA) issued a definitive position document on benzene that enumerated the risks from dermal absorption.[14]

6. SOLVENTS

Some solvents penetrate the skin even more readily than does benzene because of their marked lipid-dissolving properties. A case that emphasizes this phenomenon for the solvent 1,1,1 trichloroethane (TCA) was published recently. It involved a forty-four-year-old woman who had worked for eighteen months as a hydraulic pump dismantler and parts cleaner. She estimated that half of her daily work involved direct contact with TCA, a highly volatile degreasing agent. Much of her exposure came from her constant immersion in solvent baths. While she wore protective gloves, she reported that they always leaked, as did her respirator. Hence her exposure was via both inhalation and skin.

When she came to medical attention, she reported tingling around her mouth and a burning sensation on her tongue. Both her hands and feet were uncomfortable, with pins and needles and cramping in her feet. It was difficult for her to stand for any length of time. Measurements of her nerve conduction rates showed marked impairment, suggesting peripheral nerve damage from the solvent similar to that of William O. Her doctor recommended that she leave her work. Two months later, her symptoms in her lower legs had improved. Four months later, her symptoms had resolved completely. Except for a lingering loss of vibration sensitivity in her big toes, she felt better and her nerve conduction tests had returned to normal.[15]

These findings were remarkable on two counts. First, the chemical in question to which she was exposed had not previously been reported to produce such extensive nerve damage. Second, her exposure appeared to be predominantly cutaneous.

Controlling Skin Absorption

From these case studies it is clear that the skin is a major route of occupational exposure for many different classes of chemicals. New studies that incorporate an estimate of the dermal penetration rate combined with lung uptake suggest that such an aggregate method is a more reliable means of predicting the true risk from occupational toxic exposures than is either method alone.[16] Several contemporary researchers appreciate the newly recognized toxicity risk from dermal exposure and have advocated that dermal exposures routinely be added to risk-assessment approaches.[17]

This decision may be critical to preventing occupational illnesses, particularly as the permissible exposures to airborne contaminants are lowered. Previously, researchers simply applied a fraction of the skin dose needed to kill half of a group of test animals (LD_{50}) as the basis for warning about occupational risk from skin exposure to noxious chemicals. As a result, health hazards from dermal absorption were appreciated for only a few groups of chemicals, including the previously mentioned pesticides, phenols, polychlorinated biphenyls, and some amines.

Some of these chemicals pose such high risks of poisoning or sensitization via dermal penetration that they are given a "skin notation" by the American Conference of Governmental Industrial Hygienists. A skin notation means that all skin contact is to be avoided, usually through the use of special protective clothing and gloves. An example of a skin notation chemical can be found among the group of compounds known as glycol ethers. These commonly used solvents penetrate the skin so readily that reproductive damage is possible after only transient exposures to high concentrations of certain types of glycols.

Skin absorption of chemicals can be a problem even when the chemical is suspended in the air in a vapor, as well as when it is in liquid form. While dermal absorption for airborne chemicals is usually insignificant compared to the amount breathed, for certain chemicals like nerve gases, dermal absorption alone can be fatal. As the recent horrendous experience in the Tokyo subway demonstrated, inhalation *or* absorption of as little as two to three drops of a potent nerve gas (sarin) on the skin can be fatal or produce protracted symptoms. Certain other airborne chemicals like methanol vapors can actually condense on the surface of the body and be absorbed into the blood circulation. Even dusts of chemicals or mixtures may dissolve in perspiration on the skin and be absorbed.

How they do this was once a matter of conjecture. Today, it is clear that once in solution, most chemicals follow a simple process of diffusion into the upper layers of the skin.[18] Once through the skin, the chemical moves into the capillaries. Both factors depend on the chemical's solubility in the lipids that are found in cell membranes plus its water solubility in the blood. Small molecules that have both fat and water solubility (a seeming contradiction met by chemicals like the glycol ethers, which have both polar and nonpolar ends) rapidly penetrate the skin *and* enter the circulation.

The rate at which the chemical penetrates the uppermost layer, the stratum corneum, usually limits how much chemical comes through the skin. If the chemical is extremely fat soluble, it may be difficult for it to be removed from the skin into the blood. Under these circumstances, the chemical may build up in the epidermis and dermis, until high and sometimes toxic concentrations are reached.

This problem may prove to be particularly vexing for public health agencies that are currently monitoring airborne spray operations of pesticides to control agricultural pests. Some pesticides that are dispersed through aerosols in particles intended for insect ingestion may lodge on the skin. In Southern California, the organophosphate pesticide known as malathion is presented in bait intended for Medfly control. Such bait particles may dissolve on the skin and be absorbed. While the pesticide has been used extensively since 1980, only in 1995 was dermal absorption fully acknowledged by the state to be the dominant route of exposure. If the skin is damaged, penetration of material can be further enhanced and trace-level exposure, comparable with that experienced by the Australian sheep dippers described above, may cause subtle neuropsychological problems.

Pharmaceutical Uses of Permeation

Obviously, the length of time a chemical is present on the skin will determine how much eventually penetrates. This fact, coupled with increasingly sophisticated knowledge about appropriate dispersants and vehicles, has opened up an entirely new market for pharmaceutical companies. Many pharmaceutical houses have recently developed products that can diffuse slowly and constantly into the body via the skin. Physicians will prescribe such drugs for skin use by placing them in disks or patches of controlled size (and hence dose) that are held against the skin surface for protracted periods. A slow and predictable rate of diffusion of drugs like nicotine or estrogen from such a patch theoretically assures control over the eventual body level reached.[19]

In these circumstances, the vehicle or suspension in which the drug is placed can determine the rate at which the drug is administered. Similarly, heat, activity, and body temperature also increase the rate of transfer of chemical into the body. But, of course, the key factor in determining when and if a person is adversely affected by skin permeation of a chemical or a drug is the duration of exposure to a sufficiently high concentration to get the chemical across the skin in toxic amounts.

Real benefits for transdermal administration of drugs have been shown for premature infants in whom extra needle sticks are anathema. Because the preterm infant's skin is exceptionally permeable, successful administration of drugs via patches has been achieved for both theophylline and caffeine,[20] both used (albeit questionably) to assist early neurologic activity or lung function.

Older techniques that relied on skin-penetrating chemicals like dimethyl sulfoxide (DMSO) as vehicles for drugs have been largely abandoned in favor of these more controlled administration devices. But even the much maligned DMSO has regained a place in the skin's therapeutic arsenal. In the case in question, a fifty-seven-year-old Japanese man with pulmonary amyloidosis as a secondary result of a systemic malignancy (multiple myeloma) was treated successfully with DMSO. Just eight weeks after continuous transdermal treatment, his pulmonary infiltrates had reduced dramatically and his lung function returned to near normal.[21]

But even with the slow-release skin patch, problems can arise. Once touted as an ideal treatment for the older adult with angina pectoris, the transdermal nitroglycerin patch has come under closer scrutiny. Recent careful studies have demonstrated that after a day or two of real benefit, the body becomes tolerant to transdermally delivered nitroglycerin. Researchers who conducted placebo-controlled trials recently made a startling finding. After treating one group with nitroglycerin and the other with harmless sugar-solution patches, the research team found absolutely no benefit from any of three doses of patch-delivered nitroglycerin compared with the control.[22] Apparently, after a single day of therapy, dermal nitroglycerin loses its effectiveness. The danger of this type of treatment is self-evident: if a patient needs real nitroglycerin in an emergency, the vasodilating effect of the drug may be ineffectual because of transdermal tolerance. In spite of this dramatic experiment, nitro patches continue to be widely prescribed.

Another concern with transdermal patches is that if the drug is highly soluble in the dispersant being used, it may stay in the vehicle and very little of the pharmaceutical will find its way into the body. Conversely, if the drug is simply suspended (and has low solubility) in the dispersant, it may never leave the patch.[23] The opposite problem can occur if the body reacts to the dispersant. Should there be an allergic reaction, the resulting damage to the skin can lead to a much higher than expected influx of product into the circulation. This problem is particularly acute for blood pressure–lowering drugs like clonidine that frequently produce dermatitis.[24]

We now recognize that the skin is a ready portal to the body for both noxious and beneficial chemicals. Dermal absorption of toxic chemicals or overdose of dermally delivered drugs pose previously unappreciated risks to workers and the public alike. To better appreciate this risk, we will take a few pages to review the history and frequency of skin disease generally.

SIX

Diseases of the Skin:
A Short History

The history of skin and disease is undoubtedly as old as humankind itself. Every culture that was self-aware came to know early on that their skin was host to a plethora of disorders, rashes, and disruptions. A seemingly endless list of discolorations, pustules, plaques, papules, warts, and tumors, each with its characteristic features and signs, can be found in almost any historical medical text from the seventeenth century on. Egyptian frescoes in the tombs of pharaohs depict classical signs of skin diseases like smallpox. The two most famous medical papyri from Egypt, the Ebers and Edwin Smith Papyri, both include descriptions of skin ailments and offer remedies that are as often cosmetic (such as for hair thinning) as curative.

Where cultures have attempted to treat skin disease, they have erred on the side of trying to correct superficial changes. Perhaps understandably, early practitioners developed topical treatments in favor of less certain and possibly poisonous systemic remedies. Many of the resulting medications were highly subjective and nonscientific, but even those of nonscientific New World cultures like the Yanomami Indians were as good as or better than those developed through the Middle Ages in the Old World. European practitioners of the fifteenth through eighteenth centuries commonly used toxic poultices of mercuric or arsenical salts or purely cosmetic treatments that might include snails, honey, onions, and wax. At the same time, medical practitioners in China had already made significant discoveries about the use of the skin for diagnostic and treatment purposes and had in hand a highly sophisticated pharmacopoeia of three thousand drugs.

It was not until the nineteenth century that Western understanding of the diagnosis and treatment of specific skin diseases eclipsed that of the Near and Far East. Indeed, by the turn of the century, dermatology was the most popular "discipline" of Western medicine. By 1900, not only did all 160 of the medical schools in the United States have a separate Department of Dermatology, but its practitioners were held in highest esteem by their peers, a standing not held by modern-day practitioners of the cutaneous arts. Indeed, at the turn of the century, dermatology was at the apex of medical practice.

Western Medicine

♨ The buzz of excitement that surrounded the practice of dermatology in the late 1890s can be felt in the following description of the Fourth International Dermatology Congress, held in Paris in 1900. Delegates who visited L'Hôpital Saint-Louis, the oldest hospital in the world dedicated solely to the treatment of skin disease, observed a flood of patients eagerly awaiting treatment. A firsthand account of the dermatology clinic included this description:

> The clinic room itself is high posted and bare. Three tables and a few chairs are its only furniture. It is large

enough for a hundred people to crowd into at a point, though the adjoining waiting room will seat six or seven hundred. Into this room pour daily from three, four, to six or seven hundred patients—children first, then women, then men. . . . Usually there are three examinations going on simultaneously, with Gaucher, or De Bourmann or whoever is on service at that particular time going from one to the other and picking out for special study a case that is obscure. Behind the chairs of the examiners are grouped the eager students, among whom will be found men from all over the world who at home would be classed not as students, but as eminent skin specialists.

The patients are disposed of with lightning rapidity. A quick searching look, a skillful moving of the finger over the lesion, and then a green card here, a red card to the next, a yellow card to the third and with perhaps two words scribbled hastily on a prescription blank, serves to dispose of the great majority of the patients.[1]

In keeping with the often unsanitary and crowded conditions of late-nineteenth-century Paris, the most common disease of the time was scabies, a distressing but never fatal arthropod infection of the skin. Among the common skin diseases recognized around that time were various skin rashes and tinea capitis, a fungal infection of the scalp better known as ringworm. This recalcitrant infection was treated in the 1890s by dermabrasion using sandpaper, followed by application of a solution of mercury bichloride.

In the late 1800s, it was dermatology that bore the brunt of sexually transmitted diseases. Syphilis, still the scourge of Europe since its introduction from the New World in the early 1490s, was so intractable and indolent that it was considered best left untreated. Paget's disease of the nipple, actually a manifestation of underlying cancer, was considered just another form of eczema. As late as 1889, dermatologists still considered this deadly manifestation of underlying illness to be a parasitic disease and treated it accordingly—with predictably bad results.

By 1892, skin manifestations of lymphoma and fungal infections were well recognized, and leprosy and lupus erythematosus, an autoimmune disease affecting the skin, were studied intensively. Other diseases, notably the "psorospermoses," were in fact diagnostic artifacts that soon disappeared from the lexicon of dermatologists. The well-known view of English dermatologist Jonathan Hutchinson that eating fish caused leprosy was finally put aside in 1892. In the same year, one of the first effective herbal remedies extracted from the mustard plant was tested against lupus vulgaris, a form of skin tuberculosis.

Tuberculosis was such a dominant disease at the turn of the century that thirty-eight different types of tuberculosis of the skin were presented to attendees at the Third International Congress of International Dermatology, held in London in 1896. So diverse were its symptoms that many dermatologists believed even lupus erythematosus, which has no infectious component, to be a form of TB.

By the first decade of the 1900s, inoculation with old tuberculin was found to be an effective treatment for TB, and some forms of rheumatism was recognized as a secondary consequence of the same autoimmune reactions that caused certain skin ailments, notably erythema multiforme.

In 1900, X-ray therapy (discovered by Roentgen just five years earlier) was in vogue. Powerful X-radiation tubes were used to treat virtually every skin ailment, from skin cancer (where it was occasionally remarkably effective) to acne, excess facial hair, ringworm, and boils. Over the next six years, treatments went largely unregulated as adverse effects tended to be delayed and secondary cancers were initially unrecognized. In spite of limitations of the field, some remarkable insights into causation were made. In 1900, leukoplakia, the premalignant skin lesion that affects the inner mucosal membrane of the mouth, was linked directly to smoking![2]

While no longer dominating the field of practice as it once had, syphilis remained a focal point of dermatological study throughout the early 1900s. The great pathologist Elie Metchnikoff successfully transmitted this disease to chimpanzees in 1903. Common skin problems like hemorrhoids, syphilitic ulcers, and acne continued to be treated with dangerous ointments of mercury salts, which could be absorbed and cause serious neurological and kidney damage.

In 1906, for the first time, adverse reactions to X-ray treatments were reported, including the appearance of prominent blood vessels (telangiectasias), but the appreciation of the full extent of skin damage from X-radiation was still years away.

The characteristic rashes of infectious diseases from smallpox to scarlet fever were well documented by this time, but dermatologists still concentrated on relatively trivial problems that were amenable to treatment. In 1907, as a sign of the increasing attention of dermatology to cosmetology, the attendees at the Congress of Dermatology were treated to posters and models heralding Schamberg's Comedo (blackhead) Extractor as one of the highlights of their tour.

In 1910, dermatologists prematurely hailed Paul Ehrlich's magic bullet, Salvarsan, as spelling the end to syphilis. Multiple treatments with this toxic arsenic-containing preparation could convert to normal a positive Wassermann test (which measured syphilis antibodies), but a true cure had to await the antibiotic era. Advances in anatomy improved the appreciation of the rich vasculature of the skin and its innervation. At the Seventh

International Congress in Rome in 1912, the highlight exhibit was a startling ultramarine dye–treated human skull prepared by Werner Spalteholtz, which showed the arteries of the skin of the head in bas-relief. Silver staining showed where microscopic fibers innervated the skin and its appendages.

In 1935, dermatology entered a new era with new conceptual breakthroughs: these included the realization that focal skin infections could herald systemic illness and that radiation therapy caused accelerated aging and damaged the skin. The roster of diseases of the skin burgeoned. A compendium of skin diseases at the time included photographs of 4,566 different disorders.

Officers coming back from the Pacific field of operations in World War II reported that more of their soldiers had to be shipped home because of skin ailments than from battle wounds. As in World War I, fungal diseases like trench foot, along with gonorrhea and other sexually transmitted diseases, were also major causes of casualties in the European theater. It was perhaps understandable then why in the 1940s, when the first effective antibiotics came into use, they were used primarily to treat wartime skin infections and gonorrhea in order to return soldiers to the front.

With the discovery in 1952 that contact hypersensitivity was a cell-mediated immunologic disorder, dermatology had come of age as a specialty that fused anatomy, physiology, and immunology. For the first time, dermatologists recognized the allergenic properties of plastics, latex, and synthetic rubber. To the relief of housewives plagued by "dishpan hands," skin specialists identified contaminants in soaps and detergents as common causes of dermatitis. Ironically, during this period, treatment of a strange migrating rash known as erythema chronicum migrans (today's Lyme disease) was perfected with antibiotics. Also during the 1950s, dermatologists discovered that cortisone treatments could "cure" almost any superficial skin disorder and vastly overprescribed its use, soon to be followed with more potent corticosteroids.

In 1962, certain rashes and cases of contact dermatitis were recognized as having an industrial basis. Other conditions such as sarcoidosis were linked to exposure to zirconium, and scleroderma was associated with chronic overexposure to degreasing agents like trichloroethylene. Studies during this period (1962–1970) revealed the cause of the vulnerability of the skin to staphylococcal infections (which were found to enter through skin pores), the sources and control of fungal infections, and more about the consequences of radiation damage. By 1965, widespread use of silicone in certain upscale, urban dermatology clinics on both coasts of the United States was common, a topic of chapter 10 in this book.

In the 1970s, rational treatment for skin disorders took a leap forward, even as the tremendous political significance of skin disease became more widely recognized. Antibiotic treatments with rifampin for skin tuberculosis were by now well established, and many of the problems of control of fungal infections that had plagued earlier dermatologists had been resolved with the introduction of griseofulvin. By the early 1970s, the burgeoning plastics and chemical industry was generating thousands of cases of contact dermatitis and other serious skin injuries. Ironically, at the Twelfth International Congress in Vienna in 1972, dermatologists were instructed on the differential diagnosis of self-inflicted skin injuries to avoid unnecessary insurance claims.[3] This emphasis continued through the end of the 1970s in spite of evidence that new chemicals, especially the epoxy resins, were especially prone to produce serious cases of contact dermatitis.

Also in the 1970s, drug allergies were better recognized for their skin manifestations, and new but questionable developments for treating intractable herpes virus infections (for example, by using a few drops of the Sabin polio vaccine) were reported. The genetic contribution to many skin diseases, such as the prune belly syndrome in which the stomach muscles are flaccid, were better appreciated by the end of the decade.

By 1982, dermatologist researchers had discovered that cytokines, chemical messengers of the immune system, could explain the uncontrolled itching of many disorders. In this same period, others discovered that psoriasis could be chemically induced by elements like lithium. A cure for herpes by antibiotics like acylclovir was also announced. And researchers discovered that photosensitivity could be induced by many new drugs, especially new anti-inflammatories. Psoriasis, previously an intractable disorder, now could be effectively treated with a combination of ultraviolet light and coal tar extract called PUVA. (More about this on page 103.)

The first inkling that the skin might have immunologic capabilities was also made in the 1980s. The recognition of a skin lesion known as Kaposi's sarcoma among gay males in New York and Los Angeles in 1981–1982 was the breakthrough that led to the discovery of the HIV organism as a cause of AIDS. The roles of growth factors in the skin, notably epidermal growth factor and transforming growth factors, which could affect surrounding cells and contribute to wound healing or carcinogenesis, were also discovered at this time.

By the early 1990s, the skin had been recognized as having a full-blown role to play in the genesis of certain immune reactions. Cortisone and its relatives—the halogenated, high-potency corticosteroids—had come into their own as the mainstays of treatment for many skin disorders. At the same time, their potent immunosuppressive abilities were better appreciated and limitations on their use were recommended. Malignant melanoma emerged as the most dangerous skin tumor, having risen in incidence every year since the early 1970s. By 1995, the role of UV radiation in inducing this often fatal skin tumor—and suppressing the immune system—had taken center stage, a topic discussed in chapter 12.

The most common disorders of the skin in the 1980s remained fungal infections, and this is still the case today. In any one year, about one in twelve persons seeks medical attention for athlete's foot, scalp ringworm, or nail fungal infections. For AIDS patients, this reality is often tragic, as uncontrolled fungal diseases that start innocuously enough in the skin become systemic and prove fatal in many cases. Acne is reported in about 7 percent of the population as a whole, with most teenagers having a bout at some time in their adolescent years. Other disorders like eczema of the hands are rarer, occurring in about 0.2 percent of the population. Atopic dermatitis, psoriasis, and the skin pigmentation disorder known as vitiligo are among the second tier of common skin disorders. Taken together, these diseases affect over three million of the American population between the ages of one and seventy-four in any one year.[4]

More Americans are affected by skin diseases than by any other ailment. If buying habits are any indication of concern, the American public is probably more preoccupied with superficial skin diseases like athlete's foot, acne, psoriasis, dermatitis, and vitiligo than with any other non-life-threatening condition. Together, the prescription and nonprescription drugs devoted to the skin constitute a multibillion-dollar industry. A personal survey of major drug chains like Longs Drugs and Raley's revealed whole aisles devoted to acne and skin care treatments, skin care products like cortisone (in two strengths), and foot care and vaginal products that include new powerful over-the-counter antifungal and yeast medications. As some of the cutaneous diseases become better recognized by consumers, dermatologists are seeing increasing numbers of patients with atopic dermatitis, psoriasis, and vitiligo, the three most prevalent and potentially disfiguring disorders. Because of their notoriety, a closer look at them is warranted.

Atopic Dermatitis

The biology of even as simple and common a disease as atopic dermatitis, the typical rash of childhood, has only recently been appreciated. New data suggests that patients with atopic dermatitis do not so much have a skin problem as a systemic immunologic problem. Between 80 and 90 percent of patients with atopic dermatitis have a family history of allergy, suggesting a common heritage of a misfunctioning immune system. This likelihood is underscored by the observation that dermatitis patients commonly have food or airborne inhalant allergies and are at increased risk of getting infected with viruses that cause herpetic lesions and warts, yeasts, and bacteria.

Atopic dermatitis is characterized by intense itching. The resulting scratching often contaminates irritated skin with microorganisms that lead to widespread skin infections. Patients with the lesions typical of atopic dermatitis commonly harbor organisms from many different genera, especially *Staphylococcus aureus*, the causative organism of common boils. But the relative ease by which the colonizing organisms take hold and survive in the skin is probably a reflection of some deeper disruption of the body's normally effective defenses. Certainly, the common treatment of repeated doses of corticosteroids, which are immunosuppressive themselves, may contribute to the facility with which lesions become contaminated. The frequency of infection in these patients suggests that along with allergies, the immune system itself may be impaired.

Psoriasis

꠸ Similar suggestions about immunologic involvement have been offered to explain the plethora of problems that psoriasis patients encounter. Psoriasis causes an intensely itchy and sometimes painful, scaly, plaquelike rash that can cover large areas of the trunk, arms, and legs and affects approximately 1 to 3 percent of the world's population. For some severely affected persons, the resulting disfigurement is akin to social banishment. When the lesions spread widely, the resulting unaesthetic appearance damages self-esteem and leads many to "the heartbreak of psoriasis." This emotional overlay makes it difficult to interpret recent epidemiological studies that show an association between alcohol consumption and psoriasis. Do people who drink get psoriasis, or does the psychic pain associated with psoriasis drive people to drink?[5] The social and economic impact of psoriasis turns out to be huge for most affected persons, a fact sorely missed by most general medical practitioners but well known to dermatologists.[6]

EVOLUTIONARY QUANDARIES

Why should so many people suffer from so disfiguring a disorder? At least some portion of this relapsing and remitting disease is genetic in nature, since psoriasis tends to run in families. But which gene is responsible for what kind of psoriasis is presently unknown. More to the point, since the disfigurement of psoriasis can be socially self-ostracizing, it is probable that afflicted persons are less likely to prove attractive to a mate—and hence perpetuate their genes. If so, then it is even more perplexing why the condition is so prevalent in the population.

Perhaps psoriasis itself has some hidden adaptive function, especially in its milder forms, that gives those who carry a psoriasis gene some kind of survival advantage. If some of the genes that predispose toward psoriasis are related to those that govern the intensity of the reaction to invading bacteria, it stands to reason that a psoriasis-like *overreaction* to bacterial skin invasion may at one time have served an adaptive purpose. By responding vigorously to the threat of attack with the elaboration of a thicker keratin layer and a richer inflammatory response, individuals with the psoriasis-predisposing genome may have prospered at a time when their gene-lacking compatriots succumbed. Some clinical data support this contention by showing that psoriasis patients do have altered T-cell populations in their skin and blood suggestive of an activated immune system.[7]

A model disease for the protective role of psoriasis is cutaneous tuberculosis. It is intriguing to note that psoriasis first came to widespread attention in the dermatology community in the mid–nineteenth century, at a time when cutaneous tuberculosis—and its subsequent systemic spread—was also prevalent. But I could find no reports of patients with both diseases. Could it be that psoriatic victims were both protected from tuberculosis and given a survival edge against its more disfiguring counterpart, cutaneous TB? Because psoriasis almost always spares the face, it is unlikely to prove as much of an impediment to the initial physical attractiveness of a mate as is the cutaneous form of tuberculosis, which produces devastating facial destruction, with bulbous nose and reddened, raised patches of skin. Any protective effect against TB from a genetically based tendency for psoriatic skin—and its immunological accompaniments—would lead to an increase in the predisposing psoriasis genotype. Suggestive evidence for such protection can be gleaned from the biology of psoriasis.

While it is well recognized that inflammation and overproduction of keratin are the major clinical features of psoriasis, it remains unclear which comes first—the overproduction of keratin or the inflammation. In the past, dermatologists generally assumed that the dramatic skin changes that lead to plaques of excess keratin are the result of an autoimmune form of inflammation in the underlying skin. In the early 1990s, this attitude was reflected in the therapy of choice for treating psoriasis, namely immune-suppressing medications. The fact that cyclosporine, an extremely potent immunosuppressive drug used to fight organ-graft rejection, proved to be among the most effective treatments for psoriasis suggests that the immune system is indeed involved. But how?

DEFENSIVE REACTIONS

The most provocative idea is that psoriasis is a visible manifestation of the skin's defense against microorganisms. This idea hinges on the fact that the natural process of desquamation, by which the skin rids itself of excess layers of keratin, may be a beneficial response that normally thwarts the colonization of the skin's surface by undesirable microbes.[8] Microorganisms like bacteria or certain yeasts may pose sufficient threats to bodily integrity that the skin evolved a means of discouraging them, simply by shedding itself faster than colonization could take root.

But if this desquamation process runs too fast, psoriasis-like changes could occur in the skin. According to this theory,[9] when yeast infections occur on the scalp, the resultant excess in superficial scaling becomes visible in the form of dandruff. When it occurs on the body proper, it manifests as prepsoriatic plaques. The fact that some forms of dandruff are treatable by zinc-containing antifungal shampoos offers tentative support to this idea. By controlling the fungus, the shampoo reduces the body's need for an exfoliative response. Similarly, the anecdotal success of antifungal creams in treating mild forms of psoriasis also affords evidence for the role of yeasts or fungi in this disease.

But the skin resists molds and yeast spores by far more powerful means, suggesting that excess shedding may not be its principal mode of defense. A natural "complement" system exists in the skin that aids in the destruction of microbes,[10] and the skin's own immune functions undoubtedly aid in controlling microbial infection, a topic to be revisited in the next chapter.

VITAMIN D AND PSORIASIS

The new direction taken by treatments for psoriasis also provides indirect clues to its genesis.[11] Ten years ago, researchers discovered serendipitously that dihydroxycholecalciferol or D_3, the precursor to vitamin D found in the skin, actually inhibits the proliferation of the fibroblast cells that contribute to skin thickening and plaques in psoriatic skin. This finding has led to psoriasis treatments based on analogs of vitamin D, notably calcipotriene ointment.[12] Calcipotriene binds with vitamin D precursor receptors in the skin to stop the proliferation of keratinocytes, the major keratin-producing cells in the skin.

These new findings, coupled with the age-old use of sunlight to treat psoriasis, suggest that the basic lesion in this disease may be intimately connected to the skin's vital function in making vitamin D. Could it be that the preferential location of psoriatic lesions in precisely those areas that get *insufficient* sunlight to make vitamin D_3 (psoriasis is found predominantly on clothed areas of the trunk) is linked to local deficient vitamin D_3 synthesis? When such regions of the skin are chronically deprived of sunlight, they may compensate by making excess vitamin D_3–synthesizing tissue, just as an underproductive thyroid will increase in size to produce the missing thyroid hormone.

BLOOD CIRCULATION

Still another model posits that the skin's vulnerability to psoriasis is linked to differences in blood circulation, since some forms of psoriasis occur preferentially in the thinnest skin over bony areas like the elbows, knees, and shins. Poor blood flow in these areas may put the overlying skin at risk for circulating microbial by-products that in turn provoke inflammation and the characteristic plaquing of psoriasis.

Whatever the final explanation for its origins, the existence of psoriasis affords a window into the skin's role in defending the body against a first wave of attackers. In fact, new data has shown that the skin may have its own defense system (more about this in chapter 7). The skin makes its own "complement," a substance that assists in breaking open invasive microbes that are first coated with antibodies by the body's primary defenses. A failure in the complement system might exacerbate psoriasis.

TREATMENT

Given the advances in conceptual understanding of its origins, it is surprising that primitive, potentially dangerous treatments continue to be used to treat psoriasis. Among the most effective and controversial is the use of coal tar and its derivatives to treat the involved skin areas. A typical treatment modality has been to coat the affected areas with a coal tar derivative known as psoralen, followed by exposure to ultraviolet light (PUVA). A moment's reflection would certainly have given pause: as we have seen, coal tars were among the very first proven human carcinogens, and ultraviolet light, even when limited to the A range, is itself potentially carcinogenic or at least co-carcinogenic. In fact, crude coal tar extracts and ultraviolet light have been recognized for decades as synergistic carcinogens in animals, clearly a clarion call for caution. But as recently as 1995, researchers from the Dermatology Service of the New York VA Medical Center emphasized the lack of proof for human cancer production after coal tar applications, as an argument for continued use of PUVA while further controlled studies were done.[13] As we will see in chapter 12, in my view any decision to continue PUVA treatments for psoriasis is likely to prove a big mistake. Both radiation-induced cancer generally and skin cancer specifically can have extremely long latencies, making the safety of PUVA unproven at best.

Vitiligo

Even where disease symptoms appear limited to the skin, a deeper investigation often reveals subtle and hidden links to other disorders. This is true of vitiligo, a surprisingly common skin condition affecting somewhere between 0.5 to 2.0 percent of the population. The only outward signs of the disease are tiny circles or blotches of depigmentation. Presently, little if anything is known about how vitiligo starts or why it affects only certain family members and not others.

Perhaps because it is such a striking disorder, false associations of vitiligo with a host of other conditions have appeared throughout the last three decades. At one time or another, vitiligo has been "linked" to adrenal insufficiency, diabetes mellitus, some forms of hepatitis, baldness, lupus erythematosus, scleroderma, myasthenia gravis, candidiasis, pernicious anemia, eczema, psoriasis, hearing abnormalities, eye diseases, acromegaly, AIDS, thyroid disease, and melanoma.[14] With the exception of the last two entries, most if not all of the listed associations appear to be coincidental.

Vitiligo seems to arise in concert with the hormonal changes that accompany puberty. When it occurs, small (roughly 1 cm) circular areas of skin completely devoid of pigmentation appear. These white spots are, of course, most dramatic in highly pigmented skin. In the past, excessive suntanning or exposure to pesticides has been associated with this disease.[15] But these exposures may simply have exaggerated the appearance of the disease, since the white spots of vitiligo stand out starkly on suntanned or inflamed skin.

The best current thinking is that vitiligo may reflect a primary failure of the keratinocytes in the epidermis to support melanin production in the melanocytes. As indirect evidence for this connection, studies show that persons with vitiligo are up to 180 times more likely to develop the malignant skin disorder known as melanoma than are a suitable group of matched controls.[16] At a minimum, this data supports the idea that vitiligo results from some disturbance in the melanocytes. Even more intriguing is the association of vitiligo with endocrine disorders of the thyroid gland. Vitiligo patients are at a higher risk of developing thyroid diseases than are the rest of the population.[17] The major stimulating hormones for the thyroid and melanocytes (thyroxin-releasing hormone and melatonin, respectively) are produced in the light-sensitive pineal gland and the hypothalamus, suggesting a common linkage.

POPULAR MYTHS

Some of the myths about vitiligo originate in the notoriety of the people who have it. Much of the public interest in this condition was piqued after singer Michael Jackson explained his overall skin lightening as a consequence of treatment of vitiligo. In the instance of individuals like Jackson, who make public appearances on a regular basis, even a relatively minor pigmentation loss may present a cosmetic challenge. Normally, if the patches of lightened skin are small enough, simple cosmetic adjustments like makeup suffice. But in a dark-skinned individual, splotches of completely depigmented areas are understandably disturbing.

In such circumstances, as in Michael Jackson's case, a process of general skin lightening to reduce the contrast with the surrounding skin may make sense. A further note of skepticism that vitiligo and not simply ego pushed Michael Jackson's choice is sounded by people who observe that none of his less popular brothers or sisters have a similar disorder: if he did lighten his skin for a hereditary disease and not just to appear more "white," why are not more family members affected?

Geneticists have recently developed a model for vitiligo that at least partially vindicates Jackson's story. The model posits that multiple genes at different chromosomal sites throughout the body's genetic repertoire interact to cause this disorder.[18]

While first-degree relatives of vitiligo patients are at higher risk for developing the condition, only about one in five will actually manifest it. Hence, it is not unusual that Michael Jackson's brothers and sisters remain disease free.

Acne

Acne is the dreaded hallmark of adolescence, the facial excrescence that causes more teenagers psychic discomfort than probably any other disease. It literally defaces its victim, often at a time when self-identity is most vulnerable. While some forms of acne are evidence of industrial exposure to chlorinated hydrocarbons (chloracne), most are the result of hormonal imbalance leading to the overproduction of sebum. This overactivity of the sebaceous glands can recur in menopause, when blood levels of free testosterone outnumber those of estrogen. Whenever it occurs, such excess sebum production can plug follicles and create microenvironments that favor the overgrowth of certain pathogens. The resulting blackheads and pimples are often more than a mere annoyance. They can lead to stigmatization and social ostracism. The need for effective treatments to control this scourge of adolescence is unquestioned. But the history of our zealotry in developing and marketing antiacne medications, particularly those that might control acne in its most disfiguring form, should give us pause.

In 1982 the Hoffman La Roche Company introduced an analog to vitamin A known as isotretinoin (Accutane) to treat cystic acne. According to textbooks of the time, this orally taken medication would usually reduce inflammation and pustules dramatically. While its mechanism of action was unknown, it was initially thought to reduce the amount of sebum produced.

At the time of its introduction, isotretinoin was known to be a potent teratogen, a birth defect–causing agent, based on over three decades of animal studies on vitamin A. Early patient experience showed that any pregnant woman exposed to the drug had about a 25 to 30 percent chance of having a defective fetus. Because the drug was so persistent in the body, even women conceiving a month or more after cessation of therapy were at risk.

The defects produced by Accutane were hardly minor: serious head and face abnormalities and heart and central nervous system defects were common. While the company marketed the drug with warnings that it was contraindicated in pregnancy, thousands of young girls of reproductive age were prescribed the drug. Its teratogenic risks were so potent that blood banks were enjoined from accepting blood from patients who had received Accutane, lest residual amounts of the drug cause birth defects in an unsuspecting transfused mother. In spite of contemporary warnings that it not be prescribed "without thoughtful review,"[19] tens of thousands of young girls received the drug between 1982 and 1988.

During this period, at least seventy-eight malformed infants were born to mothers who used the drug.[20] In spite of this ongoing disaster, Accutane continued to be marketed, driven by intense demand. Accompanying warnings spelled out the necessity for patients not to conceive during treatment. But the effectiveness of the warnings and required restraint was not evaluated until 1993, a full decade after publication of the first admonition against pregnancy while on Accutane. In the interim, only a package insert and a "Dear Doctor" letter warned providers about the extreme dangers of pregnancy while on the drug.

In 1988, the Food and Drug Administration held hearings on the continued marketing of the drug. The dermatologists and company representatives present argued effectively but perhaps disingenuously for its continuation by citing anecdotal reports of suicide attempts of patients with untreated cystic acne.

In 1989, as a compromise, the FDA required a special pregnancy prevention program to minimize the risk to unborn fetuses. While this program has been remarkably effective in informing patients about the risk of becoming pregnant, some 402 women (out of a total of 122,582 at risk) from 1989 to 1993 *still* became pregnant while on the drug.[21] Of this number, most (some 270) elected to abort their pregnancies, but 32 gave birth. Given the known risks involved with Accutane therapy and the purpose of this study, it is remarkable that less than half of these infants (13) were examined for birth defects. Seven of these were found to have major or minor defects, but in only five were the abnormalities those usually associated with therapy. The resulting birth defect rate was 38 percent.

Both the dermatology profession as a group and the manufacturer clearly consider this continuing risk of teratogenicity acceptable, a fact underscored by a favorable editorial in the *New England Journal of Medicine* in July 1995.[22] In my own role in this debate as an adviser to the March of Dimes, I argued in 1991 that the trade-offs for allowing Accutane to be marketed are too extreme and that the drug should be withdrawn. My views and that of a minority of advisers were overweighed in testimony by the March of Dimes medical director and other physicians, who argued that this drug played an "irreplaceable role" in the fight against cystic acne.

Without trivializing the stigmatizing effect that disfiguring cystic acne can have on the psyche, could we not educate the at-risk teenagers about the dietary precursors to this skin condition and encourage the pharmaceutical industry to find safer substitutes for Accutane? The fact that we continue to allow this known teratogenic drug to be prescribed underscores our obsession with facial appearance and the skin.

Skin Cancer

In preindustrial England, young boys were often used as chimney sweeps. It was common for the soot and tars of incomplete combustion products to dirty their skin and clothing. A fluke of skin anatomy assured that one particularly vulnerable region of their bodies not only had chronic exposure to soot, but also was one where hygiene was most difficult: the scrotal area. The intricate folds of the scrotal rugae, as we saw in chapter 4, are ripe for chemical insult. This vulnerability is a result of their many interstices and thinness, coupled with their proximity to an underlying tissue with few if any immunologic defenses. We now recognize the scrotal area as one where chemicals can both concentrate and readily enter the body.

In 1775 Sir Percival Pott, a London surgeon, reported that young chimney sweeps were developing scrotal skin cancer in epidemic proportions. In his words, ". . . this cancer seems to derive its origin from lodgement of soot in the rugae of the Scrotum."[23] But 140 years elapsed before anyone could duplicate this percipient observation in a controlled setting. In 1915, after two years of daily painting of the skin of rabbits with coal tar, two Japanese researchers jubilantly announced to the scientific world that they had finally produced skin cancer![24]

Even though the effects of the chemical were local, it is now clear based on animal models that the active ingredients of coal tar readily cross the skin barrier and produce profound immune depression in chronically exposed individuals. Some thirty years more had to elapse before these ingredients of tar were isolated by Boutwell and his British colleagues by following the fluorescent fraction of coal tar to its logical end. Among over forty different coal tar compounds, the major carcinogen now appears to be benzoapyrene.[25]

Contemporary trends in skin cancer rates provide a critical window into possible changes in our environment. As the first tissue in contact with many carcinogens, the skin (along with the lungs) provides a kind of early warning system of environmental contamination with carcinogens. Since some of these carcinogens can interact synergistically with the ultraviolet radiation of sunlight, I have believed that it is extremely revealing that melanoma as well as the rates of other skin cancers have soared in recent years.[26] Like the canary in the mine, these tumors may be sentinels for the presence of environmental contaminants as well as the excessive amounts of solar radiation.

Studies conducted at the National Cancer Institute show that among white men, nonmelanoma skin cancers increased 60.3 percent between 1979 and 1991. In 1992, 2,100 persons in the United States died of these tumors. Most of these deaths were attributable to squamous cell and basal cell cancers. Kaposi's sarcoma, a tumor that has shown up increasingly in patients with AIDS, probably accounted for at least that number, but causes of death from AIDS have been notoriously inaccurate in specifying the contribution of any one disease process.

Given the usual stability of cancer rates over the last five decades, the increase reported for melanoma—an incredible 812.5 percent—is by far the largest increment recorded for any cancer type.[27] This explosion of melanoma cases clearly qualifies as an epidemic. While most researchers attribute virtually all of this increase to solar exposure (see chapter 12),[28] the possible contribution of chemical carcinogens to this problem should not be ignored. This is so because animal models of skin cancer have consistently shown that certain carcinogenic chemicals can work synergistically with UV light to produce melanoma.

Our modern-day environment is characterized by increased levels of UV light through ozone depletion and higher background levels of known chemical carcinogens (often the result of hydrocarbon combustion). As such, this mix is a deadly formula for cancer production in the skin. The statistics for skin cancer, and especially melanoma, which continue to soar upward, are a bellwether for disaster. If we keep on our present course, it is likely that the present upward surge of skin tumors will reach epidemic proportions both in countries like Australia and New Zealand, where a large proportion of the population is Caucasian and solar exposure tends to be intense, and in the industrialized North, where chemical carcinogens are ubiquitous environmental contaminants.

To better understand our vulnerability to these agents and how we may protect ourselves from their damaging effects, we need to understand the defenses that reside in the skin itself.

SEVEN

Bolstering Skin Defenses

For all of its anatomical limitations, the skin is a remarkably effective first line of defense against disease. We would be at the mercy of our daily encounters with pathogens but for a remarkable system that equips the skin with a germ-inhibiting barrier. This so-called acid mantle of the skin's outermost layer is an effective solution to most passive bacterial invasions. Within the skin itself is a second line of defenses constituting a previously unrecognized antigen-processing system. The skin also has a third line of defense for chemicals that transgress its outer borders: its own chemical detoxification apparatus. And deep within the skin itself are enzyme systems that permit repair of the DNA damage from ultraviolet light.

These last three bastions of defense provide a modicum of protection against all but the most severe environmental incursions. By offering us protection against damage from invading microbes, chemicals, and radiation, the skin provides us with a dramatic "edge" against the external world. The least well appreciated among these is the skin's detoxifying system.

Chemical Barriers

The first questions a toxicologist like myself asks are, Why should the skin have a detoxifying function all of its own? Could it not count on the body's primary, liver-based defense system to assure its integrity? As logical as these queries seem, perhaps we are asking the wrong questions. First, keep in mind the liver's location. If the skin had to await the activity of an internal organ to detoxify chemicals, it might itself be in peril long before the needed neutralization occurred. Second, to restate the obvious, the skin is at the body's farthermost edge and hence represents its outermost perimeter for protection against chemical and microbial invaders. Third, what passes for an "imperfect" barrier to the entry of agents from an intrinsically hostile world may be intentionally so. As we saw in our discussion of permeation in chapter 5, many chemicals readily pass into and through the skin on a regular basis.

This apparently "easy access" of chemicals to the skin's interior may be a Trojan horse adaptation. Chemicals may be let in so that they can be detoxified. Many toxic natural molecules that penetrate the skin are rendered harmless there, before they enter the body's circulation more widely. Beneath the skin lies a sophisticated chemical and immunologic defense system that permits it to metabolize and detoxify many of the most noxious chemicals that we encounter.

The skin's abilities to convert noxious chemicals, especially those with nitrogen-bearing amino side chains, into innocuous, water-soluble metabolites augments activities that at one time were considered the sole province of the liver. Like the liver, the skin contains the subcellular bodies known as microsomes that contain detoxifying enzymes. Called P-450 systems, these enzymatic batteries break down hazardous chemicals and increase their solubility in water to permit their excretion.

Among the most potent enzymes are those known as acetyl-transfereases, which can break down chemicals as diverse as the common sunscreen para-aminobenzoic acid (PABA), some highly penetrant azo dyes, and the local anesthetic benzocaine.[1] These reactions are what account for the limited, local action of sunblock creams, the loss of pigment in some tattoos, and the sometimes too short activity of topical anesthetics applied to the skin. At other times, these enzymes ensure that a drug precursor is converted to its active form. When cortisone is put on the skin to reduce inflammation, few people realize that the skin's enzymatic defense system is what changes the cortisone to hydrocortisone, the active molecule that does all the anti-inflammatory work.

A healthy skin also handles the process of detoxifying other major chemical threats to bodily integrity with such aplomb that many potentially toxic chemicals are not even perceived by the body as a whole. Sometimes, of course, the system goes awry or fails outright. This can occur when certain plants release chemicals that bond tightly to skin proteins before they can be detoxified. In the case of poison oak and ivy, this binding creates novel antigens that elicit a powerful antibody response. The resulting antigen-antibody reaction triggers an intense release of histamine that causes blistering and itching or, more rarely, an overwhelming release that dilates blood vessels and swells tissues.

Perhaps the most annoying and ubiquitous skin reaction of this sort is the one to latex. Up to 7 to 10 percent of all health care workers, and a significant proportion of the population generally, has become allergic to latex rubber.[2] When reactions ensue, as I saw recently in the case of a former nurse who went in for a simple barium exam, they can be fatal. In this case, the woman had previously developed a skin allergy to latex gloves. During an otherwise routine operation, she developed shortness of breath and dilation of blood vessels and finally collapsed and died as a result of an anaphylactic shock reaction to the tiny amount of latex in the cuff at the end of the barium delivery tube.

Reverse Effects

🖎 Paradoxically, in the course of this normally effective biotransformation of toxic chemicals, the skin sometimes fails to detoxify a chemical properly. When this occurs, instead of protecting the skin and the rest of the body from noxious invaders, the skin's "detoxifying" system creates a greater risk of damage. One striking example is the conversion of benzoapyrene, the first known polycyclic hydrocarbon carcinogen, from a relatively benign to a potent carcinogenic, epoxidelike chemical.

Repairing Faulty Enzymes

🖎 Researchers today hope that some of this well-intentioned but flawed chemical transformation activity in the skin can be thwarted through use of innovative drugs. One idea is to use a drug that inactivates the "traitor" skin enzymes. A research team at the Western Reserve University in Cleveland has isolated one from a substance found in nuts, vegetables, and tree bark that selectively inactivates one of the miscreant enzyme's activity.[3] Another drug that appears particularly promising in reversing the skin's carcinogen activation system has been isolated from Chinese green teas. But once again, researchers must be cautious in trying to manipulate the body's natural chemical machinery, because what cures one problem may create a vulnerability to a host of others.

David Bickers of the Western Reserve dermatology group has proposed that the skin's defenses might be reinforced by encouraging the skin to make an enzyme that could detoxify virtually *any* noxious chemical agent. Were this idea to reach scientific fruition, it might be possible to head off a possible industrial episode from dermal absorption of chemicals by reinforcing the detoxifying metabolic gate in the skin.

Immunologic Defenses

The concept of an independent skin system that carries out immune responses is a new one. As we saw with detoxification, physicians have long regarded the skin as a passive covering lacking in functional activities of its own. When the skin "got sick," it was considered a local affair brought on by environmental forces or local infections. Starting in about 1950, the idea that the skin was subject to immunologic damage from elsewhere in the body gained prominence. By 1960, many previously unexplained skin rashes and diseases were recognized as primarily immunologic disorders originating inside the body proper. Among these conditions were atopic and contact dermatitis. As we just learned, these conditions are primarily the result of immunologic reactions directed against skin proteins or chemically altered cellular components.[4]

But some of these reactions are the result of the unique way in which the skin *itself* handles foreign materials, be they novel proteins (as in poison oak) or metals that bind to skin proteins. Itches are the result of *local* histamine release, and contact dermatologic problems are as much a result of a local reaction to

the offending chemical as they are to the eventual systemic reaction that ensues weeks later. Among the rash of rashes that
occur in the skin, the majority probably arise from reactions
within the skin itself. In fact, the plethora of immunologic
problems that are manifest in the skin all point to a previously
underappreciated truth: The skin itself contains many if not all
the components of an immune system!

The Skin's Immune Abilities

From an evolutionary viewpoint, it is only reasonable to
expect the skin to defend itself. As our front line of defense, it
has to have a wide array of defensive strategies. One way to accomplish this defense is for the skin to have its own lymphoid
system. In 1970, a medical researcher named J. W. Streilein
postulated that the skin had a built-in, albeit primitive version
of an immune system.[5]

Originally he thought that such a system might be limited to
identifying and eliminating damaged epidermal cells.[6] Indeed,
the skin's immune apparatus is less complex than is the internal
immune system. By itself, the skin's immune apparatus probably is incapable of producing all of the reactions needed to ensure destruction of a foreign agent or organism following skin
contact. But the newly recognized array of immunologically
competent cells found in the skin suggests the presence of a
highly integrated immune apparatus. While we still do not
know fully how this system participates in the defense of the
body from pathogens and other injurious agents, some of its
functions have recently become evident.

Aberrant Cell Control

🖎 As the body's interface with the environment, the skin has to deal daily with a plethora of parasites and other potential pathogens as well as deviant cells within its own confines. Given the intense selective pressures to control cancer and keep various parasitic diseases at bay, it should not have come as a surprise that the skin itself might marshal a complex local array of cellular responses to possible parasitic assault rather than wait for the body's more distant and slower response.

But a surprise it was when, in 1983, two independent groups of investigators reported the first evidence that cells of the immune system actually lived within the skin proper. In two back-to-back papers in the same journal, these research teams discovered cells bearing a marker of one form of the cellular arm of the immune system right in the epidermis itself.[7] These cells, known as T_h-1, or T-helper 1, cells, are highly active. They can seek out and destroy foreign cells and eliminate indigenous ones that are infected with viruses or other parasites. Sometimes hyperactivity of these cells can be harmful, especially in pregnancy. Women who have recurrent abortions have been found to harbor many more of the T-helper 1 type of cells directed against the fetal trophoblast than do women with normal pregnancy outcomes.[8] In 1983, the discovery of T cells in the skin clearly implied the presence of immune competence in the skin. But histological clues for the existence of an immune system in the skin have been visible ever since anatomists looked through a microscope.

The Skin's Immune System

  Long ago, the rich network of lymphatics and blood vessels that undergird the skin should have clued anatomists that the skin was more than a passive organ or heat exchanger. This rich investment with lymphatic vessels that course around and through the dermis provides a ready network to carry soluble chemical messengers into the body proper and to deliver "processed" foreign antigens to draining lymph nodes. Within the dermis are vast numbers of cells, including lymphocytes, migrant leukocytes, mast cells, and tissue macrophages that qualify as integral parts of any immune apparatus. The skin clearly has an armamentarium of critical and competent cells equipped to handle most of the challenges that confront any immunologic apparatus. The key question was: How did these cells get to the skin? If they merely migrated to the skin from elsewhere in the body, they would not constitute an indigenous strike force any more than do U.S. troops in Bosnia. But if they resided in the skin, they would count as a native force. And that appears to be the case for at least two cellular types: specialized T-lymphocytes and immunology-active melanocytes. Together, these cells constitute a primitive immune presence in their own right.

These cells assist the body in recognizing and destroying aberrant cell types that might go on to become malignancies. In 1968, using high-powered light microscopy, I saw lymphocytes mass under new tumors and infiltrate them during a process of immune-mediated rejection. This observation was the first proof of the existence of an immunologic surveillance system within the skin that keeps skin cancer at bay.

Cytokines

☙ The skin also contains chemical messengers called cytokines that modify the immune response. When there's a breach in the skin's outer defenses, keratinocytes and other specialized cells release a flood of cytokines into the blood. This early warning system activates and mobilizes the body's immune system and draws the essential cellular fighters to the site of cutaneous injury or insult.[9]

One cytokine, known as IL-8, is probably the most important chemical mediator of our defensive network in the skin. It recruits inflammatory cells or kills invading cells outright, like those of the common yeast pathogen *Candida albicans*. In certain skin diseases like psoriasis, where an overabundance of inflammation is the hallmark, IL-8 also appears to be a central element of the body's aberrant defensive response.[10]

Keratinocyte Activity

☙ The ubiquitous keratinocytes that we visited in chapter 3 as the key producers of the surface skin keratin are perhaps the most potent accessories to the immune system of the skin. By storing and releasing its own set of cytokines, keratinocytes encourage the migration and proliferation of T-lymphocytes in the skin. Through this and related secretory activities, keratinocytes can play a key role in assisting the local immune response.

Taken together with the broader array of skin cells, it is now clear that the keratinocytes constitute an armamentarium that supplements our "front line of immune protection" against environmental toxicants and potentially pathogenic microbes.[11] How much and when these cells are called forth is still unknown. But we can infer much from experiments that alter their function. We do know that when these cells are damaged or destroyed by UV light, little or no recognition of potentially aberrant or antigenic cell types is possible (see chapter 12). This is so because any antigen that enters the skin, be it a fungal or bacterial protein, remains unrecognized by the immune system unless and until one or more of the resident skin cells takes in the material and breaks it down into smaller proteins that can be recognized by immune cells. The antigen-processing cells that do this are called the Langerhans cells.

Langerhans Cells

The Langerhans cell is at the apex of this complex mix of cells that coordinate skin reactivity. Named after its discoverer in 1868, Paul Langerhans, a German medical student, this cell type showed a remarkable ability to take up materials, like gold, that were injected into the skin. Long thought to be little more than curious histological artifacts, Langerhans cells were only belatedly (in 1982) recognized as an integral part of the body's immune apparatus. Originating in the bone marrow, these macrophagelike cells migrate to the skin and mucosal membranes, where they make up some 2 to 4 percent of the resident cellular population.

Although scattered widely throughout the epidermis, each Langerhans cell extends multiple thin, fingerlike processes, greatly expanding its surface area within the epidermis. The resulting web of extensions creates a kind of immunologic net or sieve through which antigens must pass. Most don't make it. The Langerhans cells intercept invading bacteria or fungi and process them in a way that permits their "presentation" to other cells of the immune system capable of mounting an effec-

tive response. Recent data show that if an appropriate population of these responsive cells is present when an antigen is presented, the initial process of an effective immune response can
occur *entirely within the skin itself.*[12] This fact may be a boon
or a bust, depending on how finely tuned the skin's immune
system is to "foreignness." When overly sensitive, the cutaneous immune system may overreact to certain proteins and
treat them as allergens, producing the frantic itching and dis-
traction of a delayed "contact hypersensitivity" we have previously visited in poison ivy or poison oak.

Unfortunate proof of the critical function of Langerhans
cells is their fate during HIV (human immunodeficiency virus)
infection. Of great concern is the fact that Langerhans cells are
exquisitely vulnerable to the HIV organism and die in great
numbers during the early infective stage of AIDS. These cells
are unwitting participants in AIDS progression and pass along
the virus or its infective core to the helper T cells before dying.
Thereafter, without a viable population of Langerhans cells,
the AIDS patient is subject to repeated bouts of fungal skin
infections.

Skin Transplantation

The most provocative clue for a cutaneous immune system
comes from research in transplantation biology. For thirty
years, immunologists like David Steinmuller recognized that
skin grafts "take" better if they are first perfused with saline. It
is now known that this saline washing flushes out contained immune cells that would otherwise intensify its incompatibility
with its new recipient. When these intracutaneous cells are not
eliminated, a foreign skin graft made from one individual to an-

other immunologically depressed one can actually begin to attack its host in a perversion of the graft rejection phenomenon known as "graft versus host" disease![13] Where these intracutaneous lymphocytes are naturally absent, skin grafts "take" much more readily. When lymphocyte-free skin is used for transplantation, like that from the foreskin of circumcised newborns, little or no immune reaction ensues. This fact may be partly responsible for the success of transplants made from an artificial skin made of foreskin fibroblasts layered onto degradable mesh developed by a company called Advanced Tissue Sciences of La Jolla, California.[14]

A penultimate proof that the health of skin and related mucous membranes is tightly linked to the immune system came from research among kidney transplant recipients. Since the skin's immune apparatus is knocked down by the immunosuppression normally involved in kidney transplantation, it stands to reason that one of its healthy functions is the control of the premalignant cells that lead to leukoplakia in the mouth's smooth lining or skin cancer more generally. Proof of this linkage has come from studies showing dramatic increases in skin cancers among immunodepressed kidney transplant patients.[15] Until recently, researchers thought that only body skin was at risk. A new study has now revealed highly significant changes in the skin of the lips.[16] Some 13 percent of the kidney recipients (twenty-one patients) had premalignant changes in the skin of their lips, compared with only 0.6 percent (one patient) of the controls. After almost six years of follow-up (sixty-nine months), full-blown skin cancers had appeared in two of the transplant recipients but none of the controls. As a kind of Faustian bargain, some long-term transplant survivors thus must face an onslaught of tumors that slip the fetters of their damaged immune systems.

An Overview

🖎 Data such as these strongly imply the existence of an immune system that at a minimum traverses the skin and perhaps exists within it. At the heart of this system is the presence of an entire apparatus geared to assisting the body in fighting off foreign invaders like bacteria and fungi and indigenous ones like cancer cells. The principal agents that carry out these functions may be produced in the skin itself and make it possible for the body to produce the inflammation that often heralds the first signs of a breach in our body's edge.

We still lack a full appreciation for the critical role that a skin defense system plays in protecting us against external threats. The clues for such a role have abounded. Indeed, we now know that several types of skin disease are the direct result of certain antibodies, generated by an overly vigilant immune system, lodging in the skin.[17] In particular, atopic dermatitis is now known to be mediated by the antibody group known as IgE.[18]

Conclusions

🖎 It may be that the wake-up call sounded by the extraordinary epidemic of AIDS will finally reactivate interest in the skin and mucosal immune system. These systems are now recognized as the first to give way in the onslaught of the human immunodeficiency (HIV-1) organism.[19] Many of the "diseases of the skin" itself can now be seen as adaptive reactions gone awry, a view that has been long in coming. As a student of pathology and evolution, I have learned that the key to understanding disease is to ask, What benefits do the reactions that appear to cause bodily damage have under normal conditions?

The skin's immune functions are clearly a powerful adjunct to the body's defenses generally. And many of the diseases that plague the skin, as we have seen in a preliminary fashion for atopic and contact dermatitis, may simply be the price we pay for eternal vigilance.

Where that vigilance transgresses the acceptable, a state of hypersensitivity may come about, the subject of the next chapter.

EIGHT

Hypersensitivity

One of the perennial mysteries of my biology is why I can never seem to be able to wear a wristwatch. Within a few weeks of putting on a new watch, the skin immediately under the watch invariably becomes highly inflamed, itching like crazy. This mystery was finally solved when I wore a Band-Aid under my new watch—*before* I got a rash. No rash. The corresponding problem for some women is a rash where they insert their earrings. The common denominator: something in the stainless-steel metal that induces a delayed but then florid skin reaction.

The mystery was solved when I discovered the same reaction to my silver ring. Unrefined silver typically has a high content of nickel, as does stainless steel, especially the so-called hypoallergenic steel used to make earring loops. It is now clear that a host of common chemicals are notorious for producing this nickel-like reaction. They are technically known as "sensitizers"—that is, chemicals and elements capable of producing the reaction known as allergic contact dermatitis. Following is a partial listing of the worst offenders:

AGENTS THAT INDUCE CONTACT DERMATITIS[1]

NICKEL	Nickel is present as a contaminant of many metals. Nickel sensitization usually occurs only when jewelry or other objects are worn in direct contact with the skin. Typical situations occur with zippers, cheap jewelry, earrings, and watches.
CHROMATES	Chromates are common contaminants in building cements and metal plating operations. Once sensitized, a patient may react to the residual chromate present in furs, paints, and leather.
RUBBER	Natural latex is the most common sensitizing product currently on the market. With the advent of increased reliance on latex gloves, severe reactions to skin and mucous membrane in contact with raw or processed latex have become more common (even death, as in the case I described in the last chapter), leading to strong efforts to find allergen-free rubber substitutes.
FORMALDEHYDE	Formaldehyde is a commonly used preservative and ingredient in products as diverse as plywood and cheap fabrics, where it is added to increase resistance to creases. It is a common ingredient of some glues and is used as a preservative in cosmetics and soaps.
COSMETICS	Preservatives such as the above-mentioned formaldehyde, perfumes, antibacterial agents, dyes, and fillers are typical sensitizers, much to the dismay of the casual user of both natural and synthesized cosmetic products.

RHUS
This is the general name given to the plant poisons found in poison oak and poison ivy and the Rhus tree of Australia. It is the most potent of all organic, plant sensitizers.

GOLD
Once thought to be inert, gold salts used to treat rheumatoid arthritis and other forms of this precious metal have now been clearly linked to contact dermatitis, perhaps because of contaminating reactive impurities.[2]

Those chemicals or elements produce their effects via the immune system. Some of the chemicals, including certain epoxies or detergent products, are primary irritants to the skin and produce an acute contact dermatitis (literally, an inflammation of the skin) in a matter of hours. Others may start a delayed, immune-mediated reaction that increases the likelihood that the next exposure to the same chemical will produce severe and florid dermatitis.

Exaggerated Responses

To sufferers of poison oak or ivy, it comes as no surprise that the skin can develop allergic reactions that lead to awful itching and rashes. And as any astute observer knows, once you have had a case of poison oak or ivy, you had better not come in contact with even trace amounts of the offending plant-released chemical again. If you do, you will experience an augmented reaction that can lead to massive rashes and systemic toxicity resulting from infections or generalized edema. This intrinsic "memory" of the prior exposure is stored in your immune system and the exaggerated secondary response is termed "hypersensitivity."

Chemicals that produce acute contact dermatitis are usually easy to identify and should be distinguished from those that produce their effects through more delayed, allergic-type reactions. Skin contact allergens usually affect characteristic areas of the body. The ears become involved from hairsprays, eyeglass frames, or metal allergens in earrings; the lips from lipstick, citrus peels, and certain toothpastes; the face from sunscreens, dusts, pollens, and cosmetics; the hands and forearms from poison oak or ivy, nickel, rubber, hand creams, and plants. These reactions may be mild and limited or severe and sometimes debilitating.

What makes hypersensitivity unique is the fact that very small amounts of chemicals that are otherwise completely innocuous to most persons can trigger a catastrophic skin reaction in others. The chemicals in question range in size and type from simple benzene-substituted molecules to complex plant proteins. The small molecular size of most of the offenders permits them to penetrate the uppermost layers of the skin, the stratum corneum. As we discussed in chapter 7, most of the chemicals that have the ability to produce allergic contact sensitivity lack antigenicity of their own and must bind first with naturally occurring skin proteins to be immunologically active. In so doing, these contact allergens render our natural skin proteins antigenic, alerting the body's immune system to the presence of a foreign substance. This newly formed foreign substance is typically a composite of the chemical plus the skin protein, and the immune reaction against it is limited to those areas that have actually been in contact with the offending chemical.

The resulting composite antigens are recognized by a group of lymphocytes that pass through the body's central immune system organ, the thymus, and are hence called "T-lymphocytes" (T for thymus). As we saw in our discussion of the skin's immune system, these T-lymphocytes interact with other immune cells in the skin, notably macrophages and Langerhans cells, to produce a state of sensitization. Once sensitized, further contact with the same chemical will provoke a florid inflammatory reaction at the site of contact. If the stimulus continues, a serious chronic skin inflammation can occur.

When a typical contact-sensitizing chemical such as dinitrochlorobenzene (a benzene molecule with two nitrogen atoms and one chlorine atom) is first applied to the skin, it produces at most a transient reddening or the mildest of irritations. At typical doses used in classic sensitization studies, such as 40 micrograms (40 millionths of a gram), no sign of this initial sensitization is normally seen. But once sensitized, a person who receives a second application a month later of even smaller doses anywhere on the body can produce a red, itchy, and swollen weal that may extend for several millimeters.

As our short review of the history of skin diseases showed, the clinical and occupational significance of contact dermatitis had gone long unappreciated. In the last decade, significant numbers of workers are now known to have lost their jobs because of permanent sensitization. These included laboratory workers sensitized to animal danders or urine and chemical workers sensitized to toluene diisocyanate. In 1984, these problems were considered sufficiently serious that an entire clinical journal called *Contact Dermatitis* was devoted to reporting findings in this field of study.

Phototoxicity

Another variant of hypersensitivity played out in the skin is a phenomenon known as phototoxicity. In a phototoxic reaction, sunlight interacts with a drug to convert it to a sensitizing chemical. Sunlight-reactive drugs are called photocontact allergens and are a common but underappreciated problem in medicine generally.

Photocontact allergens are chemicals that sensitize persons so that reexposure to the offending chemical and sunlight produces a classic contact dermatitis. The skin reactions are limited to those areas that are sun exposed, providing a valuable clue for the dermatologist. Typically, photosensitivity reactions are distributed around the eyes (but not the eyelids), the forehead, and the cheeks, often showing a clear demarcation where sunglasses and/or clothing have protected the skin from UV exposure. Pharmaceuticals as diverse as tetracyclines and anti-inflammatories that concentrate in the tissues of the skin generate phototoxic reactions.

In phototoxicity, it is thought that the ultraviolet ranges of sunlight produce highly reactive types of oxygen molecules that attack proteins in the membranes of skin cells and thereby create new antigens. When drugs like the quinolone antibiotics are present, they tend to block the natural enzyme systems present in the body that would otherwise protect skin proteins from damage by scavenging free oxygen molecules. The relatively low prevalence of such reactions should be cause for some reassurance, since only a handful of people who receive prescriptions for the potentially photosensitizing antibiotics develop a reaction sufficiently severe to be reported to the FDA.[3]

Much of the reactivity of the antibiotics is the result of the antibiotic chemical itself being broken down by light energy into more toxic by-products. Why this event went largely unnoticed during the premarket approval process for these drugs is in part a result of a predictable laboratory artifact: when administered experimentally to animals, test drugs rarely if ever see the literal light of day. Since all animals are caged in virtually lightproof housing and largely shielded from ambient fluorescent light, there is little opportunity for photosensitization to occur. When these reactions are provoked intentionally, they are accompanied by degeneration of the cells at the skin's surface, followed by damage to dermal tissue underneath. In experimental animals, photosensitization has been known to produce swelling and inflammation that persisted and worsened to the point of the death of the involved tissues.

Most interestingly, the photosensitization observed in test animals almost always involves pigment-free white mice. When pigmented animals are tested, they show markedly less skin inflammation than do their albino counterparts.[4] Indeed, most humans are protected from phototoxic reactions by the presence of ample amounts of melanin in their skin and the retina of their eyes.

Contact Dermatitis

As we have seen, contact dermatitis normally occurs when certain chemicals are converted to highly reactive, antigenic molecules that generate hypersensitivity. Most dermatologists who observe the characteristic distribution of a photosensitivity or hypersensitivity problem tend to treat it as a simple contact allergy, offering topical steroid creams. In practice, unless the reaction is particularly severe and incapacitating, few dermatologists concern themselves about the precise cause for reactive dermatitis and instead typically prescribe corticosteroids or related treatments that dampen the inflammatory reaction. But basic dermatology texts remind their readers of the importance of "patch" testing to determine the actual cause of such reactions.

This common medical practice of treating symptoms without identifying causes is especially troubling in the case of contact dermatitis. In its often exquisite vulnerability to offending molecules, the skin is telling us something. While sometimes annoying and rarely disfiguring, contact dermatitis reactions are scientifically revealing: they are reminders that there is a system in the skin that can break down toxic molecules into smaller, more reactive chemicals that react with skin proteins.

Adaptations

This ability of the skin to change certain chemicals into antigens that bind tightly with skin proteins was likely part of an earlier evolutionary adaptation to detoxify skin poisons right at the portal of entry. As such, contact dermatitis is both an evolutionary boon that may have served critical functions in our not so distant past and a peril, once this adaptation was "recognized" by other living species.

In this latter light, it is clearly a survival advantage to any plant like poison oak or ivy or, in Australia, trees of the *Rhus* genus to produce a skin reaction that is so discomfiting that it discourages continued eating by a mammalian host. And "mammal" is important here: unless the offending species can *learn* to recognize the characteristic shape or smell of the chemical toxin–producing plant that produced the delayed irritation, it is likely to go on blithely eating it in spite of a reaction that flares up some two to six hours after it has brushed against, bitten, or consumed the offending plant.

The existence of a mechanism in the skin for developing hypersensitivity to some substances is clearly beneficial. One need only think about the role of hypersensitivity in keeping certain yeast infections in check or in reducing the ability of parasites to gain a foothold (one should say skin-hold) in the body. In both instances, the existence of hypersensitivity reactions is "good" in that it affords protection against initial invasion and subsequent growth of dangerous pathogens.

Clearly, too, evolution has generally prepared animals to deal with chemicals that might be made more toxic in the presence of sunlight. The presence of heavily pigmented cells in the skin and retinas of virtually all animals (with the exception of the rare few who have albinism) affords good protection in the skin and complete protection in the pigmented eye against photoallergy. And too, these contact hypersensitivity reactions tend to fade with aging.

Diminution of function with age can be taken as indirect evidence for an earlier adaptive function for the skin's composite immune and nervous system. Applying this test to hypersensitivity and inflammatory reactions is revealing. What was once a rapid inflammatory and hypersensitive response to chemical irritants in the prime of youth fades significantly with age, putting the elderly at risk for developing serious skin and systemic damage from exposure to chemicals that would otherwise announce their presence with a strong inflammatory response.[5] Instead of the redness that signals an irritant, the elderly are liable to tolerate a harmful chemical with virtually no skin reaction but serious systemic consequences.

Treatment Modalities

Treatment for hypersensitivity reactions or contact sensitivity in the skin has concentrated on a single therapeutic modality: cortisone. These treatments, which include topical and sometimes systemic corticosteroids, are usually effective if a potent enough steroid is used. But the most effective steroids have undesirable side effects. Often, conservative treatment is more desirable.

For patients who have mild forms of acute contact dermatitis, the reaction will usually subside in two to three weeks with continued avoidance of the precipitating cause. Poultices of teabags, oatmeal baths, and cold water usually suffice to keep reactions in check. For more seriously affected patients, some dermatology texts recommend systemic steroids like prednisone. But these drugs have their own toxicology. Prednisone must be tapered off over a three-week period. If medication is stopped too early, symptoms may rebound. Moreover, powerful psychological effects and mood swings from euphoria to depression are common with this potent steroid, leading to dependency in some patients. Prednisone is also an immunodepressant.

More immediate, topical treatments of creams or lotions are often good treatments for the dermatitis that accompanies irritant exposures, with good old salt water (sterile normal saline) being effective in most instances. In severe cases (I once had systemic poison ivy as a result of burning the weed), bed rest in a cool dry environment is the best treatment, coupled with soaks with oatmeal or other emollients. Above all, as every mother has scolded, "Don't scratch!" (Scratching and rubbing can infect the inflamed skin, leading to severe infections.) In spite of warnings about overuse (no more than three to four applications daily), many parents overapply cortisone creams for treating their children's skin rashes. For those caused by contact dermatitis, typical over-the-counter dosages (0.5 to 1.0 percent) applied locally will not be enough, and parents are tempted to spread the corticosteroid cream over a wide surface of the body. This is likely to be a mistake.

The ability of cortisone, or specifically hydrocortisone, to control a host of skin diseases ranging from the mildest inflammations to full-blown eczema has made it a mainstay of therapy for over forty years, but too few realize that the dermal barrier readily permits this potent medicine to permeate and enter the bloodstream. Especially when used in children, it is now widely recognized among dermatologists that the systemic absorption of cortisone is fraught with danger.[6]

Although the skin-thinning side effects of cortisone are rarely seen in children, overuse of cortisone in youngsters can produce serious side effects. Should a child be treated over a large portion of his body, as might commonly be done to treat a bad case of poison ivy or oak, he or she will absorb a significant part of the dose delivered to the skin, with potentially serious hormonal or immunologic consequences. While warnings to this effect appear on all over-the-counter cortisone creams, they may not be noticed by an anxious parent. Chronic treatment with prescription cortisone creams can interfere with the nightly spurts of growth hormone so necessary for normal childhood development. The resulting stunting of growth can be a mystery, unless an observant clinician makes the connection with cortisone. The immunosuppressive effects of corticosteroids may be another problem. The more potent derivatives of cortisone can also produce characteristic water retention and distort facial features so they become bloated and moonlike, a condition known as Cushingoid features, from the adrenal steroid disease known as Cushing's syndrome.

In the future, it is clear that we will have to take contact dermatitis and its relative, delayed hypersensitivity, more seriously. The proliferation of highly skin-reactive chemicals that occurred with the introduction of epoxies and precursor chemicals of plastics and polymers like polyurethane has produced an epidemic of rashes and serious cases of dermatitis among cosmetologists and chemical workers alike. Unless we take action similar to that in Europe and more occupationally aware countries in Scandinavia, we will have to await the occurrence of still more cases of contact dermatitis before a chemical re-

ceives a "skin notation." In Germany, the notification procedure for chemicals that may pose a risk of contact dermatitis is
straightforward: under the Chemical Act, any new chemical
that is produced in excess of 100 kg/year must be subjected to
a sensitivity test in animals that will reveal its likelihood of
producing skin sensitization and must be labeled accordingly.
Similar legislation currently mandates such testing for the European Union more generally.

We now know that contact sensitization can persist long after the antigenic insult has passed. This is so because the resulting immunity becomes systemic. In fact, the superficial sign
of contact hypersensitivity, its florid contact dermatitis, is a
bellwether of an internal change that has occurred in our immune systems generally. The reality is that the skin serves the
body as the equivalent of a roadside sign, announcing to the
world that something has changed within.

A plethora of signs and symptoms of serious illnesses are
etched on the skin's surface. Many cultures have recognized
those signs early in their history, both because of their astute-
ness and because they established a historical record that
memorialized what skin changes mean. The skin is host to a
wide range of such signs, the topic of the next chapter.

NINE

Skin Signs of Illness

The modern view of the skin takes it beyond its role as a simple wrapping of the body. Contemporary diagnosticians and laypersons alike recognize that the condition of the skin mirrors inner wellness—or disease. Its role in diagnosing disease has only recently been reaffirmed. In the words of one author, few new internists recognize that the skin is a window to the internal components of the body, "the glassine [transparent] bag through which physiologic and chemical changes [of the body] are perceived."[1]

Some of these changes are self-evident. For an adolescent going through pubescence, the skin displays all too vividly the turbulent hormonal fluxes of sexual maturation. Even as an adult, the skin's condition can reflect our underlying psychological and emotional states as clearly as a road map. Anyone who has gone through a particularly trying emotional period knows that stress can be manifest in certain skin changes. Facial acne, excess oil, and perspiration all come hand in glove with psychological upheaval and personal stress.

But it is on a deeper level, where skin rashes, blemishes, and disorders reflect internal disturbances in the body's basic ability to maintain order, that the real drama of the skin unfolds.

The Skin as a Mirror of Health

✍ The fact that the skin can signal bodily illness is a common theme in folklore throughout history. Every culture has its nursery rhymes or common tales that warn children or parents of the things to watch for as signs of an impending illness. The too red face of hypertension; the exquisitely painful, swollen big toe of gout; the pallid face of sorrow or mourning. Sometimes the message is clear and urgent: A rash with bleeding under the skin coupled with a stiff neck may signal an attack of spinal meningitis. Indeed, Western medical practitioners have devised a whole registry of skin symptoms that can be used as diagnostic markers of illness. Fully five single-spaced pages are devoted to such signs in the current *Cecil Textbook of Medicine*.

Eastern Systems of Medicine

✍ What is less well known is that many Eastern medical systems have long relied almost exclusively on the skin as a diagnostic tool. In ancient Chinese medicine, the skin's surface was a mirror of internal harmony or disorder. In the centuries before Confucius, Chinese medical practitioners routinely looked to the skin for signs of systemic illness. Later, Japanese and Tibetan medicine also developed categories for illness and diagnostic systems that depended on the notion that the condition of the skin reflected the internal workings of the body. According to a fifth- or sixth-century A.D. Japanese saying, "The skin is a mirror of the internal organs."

Both the Chinese and Japanese still believe that the skin is not merely a vague mirror of the soul, but a real road map for the organs within the body. Each organ has a manifestation

along lines of force on the body's surface known as the meridians. The origins of this arcane doctrine have been connected by
the late great sinologist Joseph Needham to the development of
a unique worldview that linked the body with the earth. For the
Chinese, the body was a microcosm of the earth in all of its major features. Thus, when they developed their science of geol-
ogy that correlated surface and internal conditions, they
established a precedent for looking at the body as an integrated
whole. In geobotany for instance, practitioners were taught
that the plants that grow on the surface of the earth reflect the
internal composition of the veins of minerals within.

Prospectors were taught that certain plants have a high tolerance for otherwise toxic concentrations of metals. Plants
growing above ground heavily contaminated by these metals
serve as a flag for the presence of lodes or deposits of minerals
with those elements below the earth's surface.

According to Needham, it was a small step from geobotany
to cutaneous diagnosis, the close inspection of surface characteristics of the body to discern the condition of the organs within.
A red rash or inflammation at an acupuncture point or along a
meridian could signal a diseased organ deep within the body.
Such a view made perfect sense to the Chinese because of the in-
terchangeability of the features of the earth and the human body.

The Buddhist prohibition against autopsy and dissection
further intensified this belief system, since it limited medical
practitioners' experience with internal pathology. Early practitioners of Chinese medicine were thus naturally inclined to
search for signs of disturbance of internal organs by looking—
very carefully—at the surface of the body. Just as the earth signals the presence of ores within by surface configurations, the
body signaled the presence of disturbances in the organs and
their interrelationship by lines and conditions at the body's

own boundary—the skin. The great circle meridian on the skin, for instance, reflects the condition of the lungs, while the intestine meridian reflects the condition of several internal organs, including the small intestine.

Signs and conditions of the skin itself were thus taken as evidence of conditions in the body and vice versa. This realization is based in part on the Chinese system of "correspondences," wherein various conditions of ill health are reflected by and interrelated to a network of organs, which in turn is related to the seasonal cycles of birth, growth, ripening, harvest, and decay. For instance, when the skin is cracked and dehydrated it signifies a condition of *Dryness*. This may simply be due to a dry climate or may reflect an imbalance between the body and the internal fluids that keep its tissues moisturized and usually means a deeper, systemic disturbance. This disturbance may be anything from diabetes, in which fluid imbalance is a dominant feature, to kidney dysfunction, in which the body fails to excrete adequate amounts of toxins like urea.[2]

To the Chinese, the meridians on the skin demonstrate the continuity and interconnectedness of the organs within by manifesting certain lines of force known as *Qi* (life energy) and surface features (the acupuncture points). The tongue, a highly concentrated piece of epithelial tissue, had the greatest diagnostic value of all. While many may decry the seemingly superstitious nature of this metaphorical doctrine, it was based on a long history of empiric medicine and clinical experience.

The Chinese practice of using the complexion and condition of the skin as a ruler for measuring internal homeostasis was advanced beyond its time. Not only did the Chinese recognize that the skin represents the first line of defense against what they called "noxious external influences," but they intuited that the skin itself contained a measure of resistance. In their lexicon, skin was considered to be the principal domain of the body's defensive energy, or *wei qi*. This prescient view anticipated the discovery of a skin-specific immune system by over two thousand years!

Homeopathic Approaches

~ Modern-day homeopaths practice a form of medicine that was developed by Samuel Hahnemann in Philadelphia in the 1800s as an alternative to the often harmful allopathic remedies of his day. Homeopathy relies on the ability of ultralow, "potentized" doses of agents to cure disease by identifying and using those substances that at high dose produce disease symptoms analogous to those experienced by the patient. Homeopaths believe that the idea of purely "skin" disease is a myth. According to Hahnemannian doctrine, each superficially visible disorder on the skin is a manifestation of an internal disturbance in the body proper. In the words of homeopath Dana Ullman, "Homeopaths do not consider skin diseases to be actually diseases of the skin; they are internal conditions which create symptoms that manifest on the skin."[3]

Just how valid and useful is this dictum? Certainly many skin ailments happen on the skin because the skin itself is injured. Rashes, warts, skin tumors, and swellings from bacterial infections all appear to be "skin specific." But in keeping with homeopathic guidance, we would be wrong to stop our investigation of all skin ailments at the surface of the body. As we saw with lupus erythematosus, a rash may signal a local reaction to a wholesale autoimmune attack on the body infrastructure.

Western Medicine

This view of the skin as a bellwether of illness was long in coming to Western medicine. For centuries after Galen offered his doctrine of the four humors, which predicted disease by noting skin coloration, Western practitioners were held in thrall by the viewpoint that the skin revealed general temperament but rarely any specific internal illness.

Even after the age of modern medicine dawned in the mid-1800s, and as late as 1900, clinicians believed they could achieve successful superficial treatment of skin ailments, even when those ailments actually signaled more widespread disease in the body. The success of Danish dermatologist Niels Finsen in curing lupus vulgaris merely by shining intense light rays on the face was taken by many as evidence that tuberculosis could be cured by heliotherapy treatments. In fact, lupus vulgaris is only an external sign of more widely distributed, systemic tuberculosis. Light treatment, while effective in removing the cosmetic blemish of this disease, did little if anything to cure the underlying illness. Even with a spontaneous "cure" of cutaneous tuberculosis in immunologically competent adults, the tubercular bacillus almost always continues to lie fallow, ready to spring forth should the immune system falter again. This message is painfully clear to many AIDS patients, who sometimes experience recurrent TB after "successful" antibiotic-mediated eradication.

The lesson from contemporary pathology is that all elements of a disease process are never evident to the naked eye. A diagnosis can be made solely by looking at the skin's surface, but what happens at the body's edge may not be the entire story. More particularly, what may start as a superficial lesion that is properly diagnosed as a skin disease can change with time.

This circumstance has no better example than Kaposi's sar-coma. Named after Moritz Kaposi, who discovered it in the last decade of the 1800s, the purple-and-red splotches of Kaposi's occurred rarely and then almost exclusively among elderly Jew-ish men of European ancestry. As we saw in chapter 1, in the 1980s a surge of new cases of Kaposi's among homosexual men was reported in Los Angeles and New York—and thereafter throughout the United States. Now the disease is recognized as a hallmark of human immunodeficiency virus (HIV) infection and may be caused by a variety of the herpes virus set loose by the body's flagging immune system. In this sense, Kaposi's is the epitome of a skin manifestation of internal illness. Indeed, the linkage of Kaposi's to the immunodepression of AIDS has suggested accurately that the original disease itself reflected a systemic immune disturbance.

Modern-Day Diagnostics

Today every dermatologist is trained to recognize the skin as a flag for internal problems. The modern view of derma-tology as a science of both diseases of the skin and the skin as diagnostic tool for looking at the body took hold in the mid-1950s. Whole texts are now written about the manifestations and signs of disease that can be signaled through changes in the skin.[4] *Cecil Textbook*'s list of diseases that are flagged by skin changes includes diseases of the digestive system, including gas-trointestinal bleeding; liver disease; metabolic disorders; kid-ney disease; and diseases associated with hypersensitivity.

The skin disorders that signal the presence of rheumatologic or autoimmune diseases deep within the body are particularly critical in making an initial diagnosis. As we saw, a simple rash may signal the presence of a deep-seated autoimmune problem like lupus erythematosus. Similarly, the blanched fingers of Raynaud's disease may be an early sign of scleroderma. In other rheumatologic problems, a skin disorder may result from the body's response to a microorganism that provokes an immune reaction that coincidentally cross-reacts with an essential body part. Other diseases have an early, passing skin sign (the syphilitic ulcer) that progresses insensibly until later disease stages signal their presence by more visible skin malformation.

Eight examples serve to underscore the critical importance of recognizing internal illnesses through their skin manifestations.

1. SPIROCHETIC DISEASES

Lyme disease, caused by the spirochete organism *Borrelia burgdorferi*, is often signaled by the presence of a spreading bull's-eye-like rash that emanates from the site of a tick bite.[5] The syphilis spirochete is another example. A chancre appears at the site of initial infection, only to disappear in two to six weeks as the syphilitic organism spreads more widely to produce secondary syphilis.

2. BACTERIAL ILLNESSES

Certain bacteria, such as the *Neisseria* species responsible for most cases of meningitis, produce a characteristic rash only *after* they have spread systemically. Then, the skin sign represents the presence of an often serious, internal disease. Similarly, the gonococcus *Neisseria gonorrhoeae* usually produces its typical, innocent-appearing skin pustule on the fingers only after gonorrhea has spread throughout the body.

3. THYROID DISEASES

In diseases of the thyroid, particularly hypothyroidism, a condition in which diminished amounts of thyroxin lead to a generalized slowing of metabolism, changes in the skin and hair are frequently the first signs that hormonal balance is out of kilter. In patients with hypothyroidism, the skin is characteristically pale and dry and the hair undergoes thinning. In extreme cases, complete hair loss (alopecia) occurs. The converse condition, hyperthyroidism is associated with a flushing of the skin, rapid pulse, and nervous tremors, reflecting the acceleration of metabolism that underlies this disorder.

4. ADRENAL AND OVARIAN TUMORS

Should acne and excess hair appear, particularly in a middle-aged woman who is experiencing menstrual irregularity, it can be a sign that the patient has a male hormone–secreting tumor of the ovaries. In a younger woman, virilizing effects that include skin coarsening and hirsutism may be a sign of an adrenal tumor.

5. CANCER AND LYMPHOMA

Another tumor that signals its presence with cutaneous signs is lymphoma. Here the occurrence of plum-colored, horseshoe-shaped patches in the skin can disclose the presence of an enlarged spleen and lymph nodes that commonly occur in lymphoma. In advanced cancers, a "carcinoid" syndrome in which the tumor itself releases a melanin-stimulating hormone can lead to a dramatic darkening of the skin. This melanotic reaction is occasionally a first and most ominous sign of a deeply seated cancer of the lung.

6. ARTHRITIC DISEASES

The skin serves as a clear marker of disease in many so-called reactive arthritic illnesses and autoimmune diseases. Rheumatic fever caused by streptococci (type A or G) is signaled by a sore throat (pharyngitis) and a classic streptococcal rash called "erythema marginatum." In this case, a well-demarcated red rash signals a more dangerous reaction to infection internally.

The full-blown rheumatologic consequences of this initial skin and throat infection are well known to clinicians: transient joint pain and antibodies that attack elements in the skin and the mitral valve leaflets in the heart. When autoimmunity persists, this skin rash and the accompanying reactive arthritis can last from two to three months, and the heart valve may be permanently weakened.

7. LUPUS ERYTHEMATOSUS

Another arthritislike illness that commonly reveals itself through a reaction at the skin surface is lupus erythematosus. Lupus manifests itself as an eruption of reddened and sometimes thickened skin over the bridge of the nose. Rheumatologists now recognize this butterfly-shaped rash as a cardinal sign of lupus, one that may indicate that ongoing autoimmune disease processes are happening inside the body. As we have seen, earlier this century, various forms of lupus were treated as if they were superficial diseases, limited to the skin.[6]

Often the presence of the rash and its severity tell the observant dermatologist not only that a disease process may be under way, but something about its severity and extent. While the skin signs and manifestations of lupus were once considered to be so diverse as to defy classification, it is now clear that the patterns of different forms of cutaneous lupus erythematosus are highly predictive of the degree of severity of systemic disease any given patient may experience. A typical listing provides twenty-six skin or mucous membrane lesions that have been reported to occur with lupus, including discoid and wart-like eruptions, butterfly-shaped rashes over the nose, psoriasis-like changes, and even squamous cell carcinoma.[7]

For some patients, a benign, self-limiting skin eruption is all that ever shows up. But for others, more extensive skin damage signals a deep, underlying illness that envelops many internal organs. This latter form of systemic lupus erythematosus can be fatal.

8. IMMUNE SYSTEM DISORDERS

Another illness that is signaled by the skin is a familial disorder known as Wiskott-Aldrich syndrome. This condition results from a defect in the immune system and leads to a heightened susceptibility to infection. One key manifestation is a common skin rash indistinguishable from classic atopic dermatitis. When Wiskott-Aldrich syndrome is treated successfully by providing a bone marrow transplant, the rash clears almost overnight. This dramatic finding was the basis for the idea that atopic dermatitis is at root an immunologic disorder and has suggested new and effective therapies for its cure.[8]

Drug Reactions

The skin is also a mirror of adverse reactions to a variety of drugs. Therapeutic agents ranging from aspirinlike anti-inflammatory drugs to gold produce typical rashes. These rashes may portend nothing more than a slight allergy, or they may signal internal reactions that may reduce or reverse the effectiveness of the drug's primary intended effects. An extreme example is the reaction to penicillin-based antibiotics. Many individuals develop an allergic reaction to penicillins as a result of repeated exposure, especially in childhood. My spouse has such reactivity, but it went unrecognized until her adult years, and even then, the recognition came almost too late. An oral dose of penicillin led to a breakout of hives that covered her whole body. Her hands swelled and her face flushed. She was close to being in anaphylactic shock, a life-threatening condition in which antigen-antibody reactions lead to histamine release, loss of blood pressure, and swelling in the throat that can cut off the windpipe. In cases of full-blown anaphylaxis, administration of epinephrine and an antihistamine may be necessary to cause the symptoms to abate and permit recovery. My wife now wears a bracelet alerting the medical profession to her condition.

Conclusions

The skin may be not so much assailed by disease itself as reflecting the presence of disease somewhere else in the body through a characteristic disfigurement or sign. Recognizing and understanding these signs requires vigilance at the body's surface. Indeed, a central message of this book is that healthy skin may be critical for our more general well-being. In recording the disruption of the skin's normal vibrant appearance, prescient observers may detect a critical early warning for an illness smoldering unnoticed deep within the body. Sometimes, a rash or papule may be the body's way of signaling that its front line of defense has been breached. At other times, it is a signal of a full-blown illness.

The Body's Scarlet Letter

In time, cultures have come to recognize some of the most common "skin signs" of major illnesses. When these cardinal signs of illness are recognized as signals of disease, they begin to acquire an evolutionary significance. Lepers are banished because of their excruciatingly visible signs of their infective status. The swollen nose of rosacea (W. C. Fields's condition) or the more florid disfiguration of lupus vulgaris usually makes their holders less attractive and thus reduces their fitness in an evolutionary sense. The purple splotches of Kaposi's sarcoma are our nation's current stigmata.

When persons affected by these and other signals of disease fail to mate and reproduce, the genes for susceptibility to their conditions die out accordingly. Where a family member with a contagious disease gave no warning sign of his illness, others would soon become infected. Elsewhere, when active disease gives a clear warning, as in measles or smallpox, steps to avoid contact during the period of greatest contagiousness are possible. Other diseases, such as lupus erythematosus, that are flagged by characteristic skin signs may also be signaling their presence to prospective suitors: "Marry me and our children may face the same life-limiting disease."

Still other rashes or papules may engender learned responses: "Stay away, I have a contagious illness." In this way, skin signs may once have provided powerful evolutionary messages. When heeded, the distancing effect of these signs may have led to the reduction of the distribution of susceptibility genes. But more often, our penchant to regard anyone with a visible deformity as disfigured and socially undesirable has led to a less salubrious moral outcome: many of the skin signs of illness have come to be taken as hallmarks for banishment and stigmatization. Smallpox is just one example. The characteristic pockmarked face of a survivor of smallpox or its weaker relative, chickenpox, was irrationally considered a mark of lower-class status and contagion. The skin signs of late syphilis, TB, and leprosy were all used at one time in history to ostracize the sick.

Today, acne is mistakenly assumed by some to reflect ill health and disfigurement, even as its effects may be local and transient. The resulting loss in self-esteem from even the slightest blemish has led to the emergence of a massive industry designed to perpetuate the myth of the necessity of pure skin for social acceptability. The apotheosis of this industry was the perfection of plastic surgical techniques that could transform the skin. One of its most potent tools is a modern-day chemical miracle known as silicone.

TEN

The Silicone Story

In the hunt to retard aging and control the natural transformation of our outward countenances, the skin has proven an elusive quarry. With time, the telltale signs of aging—wrinkles, sags, and frown lines, in particular—are captured indelibly on our faces. But acceptance of the inevitable is rarely the American way. In the last forty years, the socially driven need to retain youth not only has spawned the vastly expanded market for cosmetics, but has fueled the emergence of the new field of cosmetic surgery.

It is the maxim of cosmetology that people can control and improve their self-image. By emulating movie greats like Cher, who successfully battled disfiguring acne as a teen and aspiring young star, we believe that we can literally "change our skin." But we soon learn that altering our appearance entails much more than wearing a night mask or changing our diet for a few weeks. What Hollywood demands is often nothing short of a wholesale transformation and the elimination of any physical defects. And the quest for this metamorphosis has on many occasions put its seekers in harm's way.

Origins of Cosmetic Surgery

🖜 Plastic surgery is the field of medicine directed at repair of physical defects. It began with Hindu physicians in 800 B.C., who successfully grafted skin from one place on the body to another to replace missing structures. Vedic treatises of the time describe how flaps of skin from the forehead were used to fashion new tissue for a sword-damaged or excised nose, often the price a woman paid for infidelity.

Its modern surgical equivalent can be traced to an Italian surgeon named Tagliacozzi, who practiced in the sixteenth century. In 1597 he described how he grafted new tissue onto a soldier who had lost his nose in battle by creating a skin pedicle from the wounded man's elbow to his face. This daunting prescription for a new nose entailed the soldier's holding a skin bridge in place, elbow to nose, for five weeks before it was cut free. We now believe that the resulting graft was successful because it retained its original blood supply from the arm while it was healing to the face.

Modern plastic surgeons initially concentrated on the repair of equally severe congenital facial defects, like cleft lips or palates, rather than on cosmetic procedures. (The first successful cleft palate operation in the Western hemisphere was performed by a surgeon named John Peter Mettauer [1787–1875] in 1827.) In such instances, restoration of a semblance of normalcy posed the major challenge to surgical acumen. Expansion of such efforts to correct less severe facial deformities, such as deformed chins or sunken cheeks, spawned the field of plastic and reconstructive surgery in the early 1900s. While the first rhinoplasty (the technical term for a nose job) was performed around this time, cosmetic surgery did not come into its own until several decades later.

With the advent of World War I, plastic surgeons were urgently needed to treat head and jaw injuries. Repair of skin defects and replacement of burned skin was accomplished only through heroic efforts, many of which failed. Twentieth-century plastic surgeons had their most dramatic successes in repairing major skin defects largely as a result of perfecting new techniques of cutting and reconnecting skin. Among the most simple and dramatic such achievements was the development of "Z" plasty, wherein skin was cut crisscross and extended to repair defects. By not sacrificing the skin's own blood vessels, success was routinely achieved as long as strict asepsis was practiced.

In 1932, when the American Society of Plastic and Reconstructive Surgeons was formed, "legitimate" plastic surgery was confined largely to assisting patients suffering from trauma-produced or congenital facial defects.[1] Cosmetic surgery, whose ends are improvement as much as restoring a semblance of normalcy, received only a grudging recognition from its more surgically inclined practitioners over the next two decades. In the 1930s, face-lift patients were perceived as going to unscrupulous surgeons, often unskilled in the arts of true plastic surgery.[2] After World War II, cosmetic surgery boomed but did not receive full recognition among the traditional practitioners of plastic surgery until the next decade.

The Cosmetic Era

Although some "nose bobs" were performed in the 1930s to "correct" profiles that appeared too ethnic for the prevailing Anglo-Saxon norm, cosmetic surgeons gained acceptability in the 1950s with the widespread use of the face-lift and surgical correction of facial wrinkles, furrows, and baggy eyes. But the effects of cosmetic surgery tended to be transitory. Sometimes, as with the "pull-back" surgery to reduce wrinkles on the forehead and around the eyes, plastic surgery left the face with a wooden, strained, or surprised expression. And as with any surgery requiring general anesthesia, such cosmetic tinkering was not without its own set of side effects, from septic infection to outright deaths from overanesthetizing patients in office settings without resuscitation equipment.

Side effects among cosmetic surgery patients were particularly severe in post–World War II Japan. Skin and tissue augmentation for new breasts, buttocks, and thighs that "fit" the new Western ideal of beauty were achieved with often heroic but ill-advised surgery and injections of fluids of uncertain and untested composition. Diverse chemicals, from paraffins, industrial silicones, and peanut oil to plastics, were injected or surgically implanted to "improve" the appearance of the Japanese physiognomy, often with disastrous results. Many women developed disfiguring skin conditions like scleroderma and irreversible autoimmune conditions from the unbridled immune stimulation brought on by paraffins and other products.

The Silicone Scene

🌲 With this history in mind, it is perhaps understandable that a whole generation of cosmetic surgeons enthusiastically embraced the news of a technology that promised to avoid these catastrophes through simple injections of an inert, biocompatible fluid. The material at issue was medical-grade silicone.

Silicones had initially been fabricated during World War II as a chemically inert, heat-resistant lubricant that could be used in the high-temperature engines of airplanes or as seals and gaskets for the temperature extremes encountered by military equipment. A derivative of these industrial products was developed in the late 1950s as "medical-grade" silicone oil. This medical fluid was actually identical to one of the original industrial silicone fluids, with the exception of some unspecified "quality control" procedures.[3] The demand for this ostensibly inert material prematurely pushed it into human application even as the parent company, Dow Corning Corporation, was conducting the first rudimentary animal trials.

In spite of the lack of long-term safety data from animals, in 1964, Dow Corning conscripted a select group of plastic surgeons to participate in an FDA-approved limited trial of human silicone injections. Dow Corning promoted its new product by asserting that silicone oil offered the cosmetic surgeon greater control over the size and shape of the resulting implant than did traditional solid implants. Dow Corning also promised that injected silicone would produce no scarring, conform to the body's contour, and provide a normal texture to the deformed features. Its safety, they stated to the FDA, "is based on the well-known physiological inertness of silicones in general and dimethylpolysiloxanes [silicones] in particular."[4] This statement was contradicted by internal studies done by Dow Chemical Company sixteen years earlier that demonstrated metabolism and irritant properties of some silicones.

Dow Corning emphasized to the FDA that the proposed studies would involve amounts ranging from 0.02 to 0.1 milliliters (for wrinkle treatment) but acknowledged that as much as 100 milliliters (0.1 liters) might be used to treat the loss of muscular and subcutaneous tissues. These amounts, according to Dow Corning, were well within the safety range of silicone, a statement unsupported by any long-range testing and actually refuted by their own testing between 1968 and 1970.

FDA Approval

When the FDA gave its initial approval to the investigational use of injectable silicone in 1965, it stipulated that the product would be used only by the Dow Corning–selected doctors and that these authorized plastic surgeons would treat only those patients who had severe, debilitating cosmetic deformities. Sale of the product itself was to be limited to ampules containing either 1 or 50 cc's (1 to 50 thousandths of a liter) of material, and the FDA urged that only low-volume injections be done. The initial treatment team consisted of seven American plastic surgeons, most with extensive practices and all with impeccable credentials within their field.

Within these guidelines, any part of the body was initially fair game for an injection procedure, but only injections of small amounts of silicone were recommended. Full-scale testing began almost immediately. In 1967, the FDA temporarily suspended testing for a year until more animal data could be gathered. From 1965 to 1966 and 1968 to 1970, the period of most active legal human testing, 973 patients were injected with silicone by the team of authorized surgeons. During the same period, further data was accrued from animal studies ranging from mice and rats to macaques and apes. In 1969, after adverse effects were seen in patients who had been injected with large amounts of silicone in their limbs, a more limited protocol was adopted that singled out defects that involved severe loss of subcutaneous tissues in the cheeks.

Testing Results

&~ Deviations from the FDA guidelines were evident in some of the initial reports of the human studies. Patients with otherwise non-incapacitating but cosmetic deformities, such as the loss of a small amount of muscle mass, were injected with tens to hundreds of cubic centimeters of silicone, far in excess of the tenths or hundredths of a cc recommended by the FDA. Adverse effects were also in evidence. Occasionally, the fluid would dissipate by migrating into more distant tissues, or it would provide a florid inflammatory reaction that caused even greater anatomical disfigurement than the original defect. Tissue reactions occurred, even with smaller injected amounts. One patient who received only a few tenths of a cubic centimeter of silicone in the furrow between her eyebrows developed a walnut-sized growth some months later.

While reports to the FDA and the medical community from the animal testing performed in the mid-1960s assured them that only minimal adverse effects were observed, the raw data from some of the reported studies showed quite a different picture. For instance, Dow Corning reported to the FDA in 1965 that the results of these studies "show that the injections were tolerated by the tissue with only minimal inflammation resulting."[5] The actual studies by Drs. T. D. Rees, D. L. Ballantyne, and Franklin Ashley showed that many of their injected monkeys and apes had significant portions of their body tissues distorted by silicone by varying degrees of chronic inflammatory changes. The raw data from the ape studies in fact provided evidence of a strong inflammatory reaction in injected tissues, along with death of fat cells and migration of silicone to other organs like the salivary glands under the jaw.

In spite of assurances from Dow Corning to the FDA that

any inflammation seen was minimal and "resolved in a short time," much of this research failed to follow up treated animals for a sufficient period to warrant this assurance. And when follow-up was done, some of it in fact demonstrated the formation of chronic inflammatory changes. A detailed look at the key study performed by Dr. Franklin Ashley at UCLA, which included rats, two Rhesus monkeys, and ten Japanese apes, would then have provided some insight into the health consequences of silicone injections made to the face and breast areas.

The Ashley ape work in particular was designed to be a definitive prototype of what was done in humans. Each animal received multiple injections of silicone into both the cheeks and the breasts. Dow Corning reported that this study found "no abnormalities in any of the animals except the local increase in soft tissue bulk in the areas of injection."[6] In fact, the original data showed that several of the treated animals, in particular one Japanese ape named Big Ben and another named Sumi, had experienced severe reactions, including what the author's notes indicate as the "complete destruction of the architecture" of Big Ben's face where injections had been made.[7] Breast tissue injections were even less satisfactory and produced encapsulations and fluid loss through migration.

The full extent of the findings of this study have never been published. As a result, neither the FDA nor the treating physicians in the human protocol were told that pathological changes occurred with even the "purest" silicone. Often, controls were minimal or omitted, so that true interpretation of data was compromised.

Findings from the concurrent treatment of human subjects were even less reliable scientifically. Of the seven initial investigators, most reported no adverse effects at all except to note that some fluid was "lost" after injection. This was particularly true if the injecting surgeon missed the tricky within-skin injection (intradermal) and instead injected silicone below the skin (subcutaneous). In other instances, astute observers noted that silicone was found to migrate to the lymphatics and lymph nodes, an ominous finding that was later to prove of greater consequence to silicone's immunologic activity. Intradermal injections occasionally led to recurrent skin reddening (erythema) that lasted for months or to "recall flares" when subsequent implants or injections were made, suggesting that allergic reactions to silicone might be occurring.

In one particularly extensive series of 711 patients injected by Dr. Orentreich, an authorized physician from New York, adverse findings were reported that should have given the investigational team pause. Between January 1965 and October 1967, Orentreich gave each patient an average of twenty-six separate injections to the face of 0.025 cc each to repair facial scarring and wrinkles. Orentreich reported that about 10 percent experienced undesirable side effects.

Because this disturbing rate of adverse reactions was not found by other, more conservative physicians on the team, it was largely ignored rather than being examined for possible applicability to the project as a whole. For many of the others who used fewer injections, patient outcomes appeared almost too good to be true. Even where different types of fluid were tried, little or no reaction was reported. At least one male human subject was injected in January of 1964 with five different viscosities of silicone oils in the midline of his back. He was observed for 3½ years. In this instance, punch biopsies of the treated areas showed virtually no tissue reaction.

The collective experience of the investigators was so good, in fact, that the FDA was suspicious. Some investigators waxed so eloquently about the virtues of silicone both before and during their trial experience as to call into question their objectivity. Many of their confidential reports warned about the dangers of injecting directly into blood vessels (at least two persons out-side the protocol died from such a result), into abraded skin, or into extremities like the penis. But their more public pro-nouncements and communications extolled the product. One authorized physician stated that "I am almost embarrassed to review eleven years' work with silicone fluid without any seri-ous difficulties to list."[8]

Adverse Effects

Others were apparently not so lucky. During this same period, at least one authorized physician described a serious problem of the migration of silicone down the leg of a patient who had been injected in October 1966 with 32 cc of silicone to augment the calf muscles of both legs. In this case, a thirty-two-year-old woman had developed recurrent inflammatory nodules and was described as being "allergic" to the silicone fluid. She developed an abnormal thyroid function test, with cysts evident on biopsy. She also developed calcifications along the tracks where the silicone migrated. Biopsies of the exposed areas showed a marked foreign body response. The patient was eventually treated with a powerful anti-inflammatory called Butazolidine, then used illegally to augment the performance of racehorses.

Like many women who allege adverse reactions to silicone, this patient was considered to be hysterical and was given elec-troshock for her fatigue and depression. Subsequently she was treated with plastic surgery to repair the damage. The resulting skin flap died and sloughed off one week later, leaving her with a major scar and deformity. Her treating physician, Dr. Edger-ton, closed his report with the strong recommendation that no one be injected in the legs with silicone fluid.

Presciently, he urged that his patient be assessed for a probable reaction to silicone injection with chronic inflammatory response, a common finding in women with ruptured silicone breast implants. This report appears to have fallen on deaf ears, since no mention of systemic side effects from any silicone preparation appears in Dow Corning's silicone literature until after it had lost its first silicone breast implant case in 1984.

But adverse reactions were not confined to patients injected in their extremities. At least one physician outside of the American program had a comparably poor outcome when using silicone fluid according to the Dow Corning design. This doctor treated the atrophied cheeks of a patient in April 1964 with 28 cc of silicone oil. The patient developed a flulike illness some 240 days later, accompanied by painful extremities, headache, low-grade fever, and tender "lumps" along the chin line. A tumorlike growth, probably reflecting an expanding granuloma, appeared on the left cheek, another a few months later on the right cheek. Neither responded to antibiotics. Whether or not this episode represented an immunologic response to silicone or a smoldering infectious response cannot be discerned from the records.

In spite of these questionable findings, by March 1972, Dow Corning reported that the results were sufficiently favorable to merit an intent to submit a formal New Drug Application by June. While acknowledging that volume loss was a problem in recently enrolled patients, Dow Corning wrote that silicone injections would be safe since they were taken into macrophage cells and transported to the lymphatics without observable ill effects. They reported that no systemic effects were seen, even though no pathology of draining lymph nodes from human subjects was available or long-term examinations for systemic illness undertaken. Ominous signs of organ damage such as elevated liver enzyme tests, were periodically observed but not followed up.

The Downside

By the early 1970s, this experiment was clearly out of control, and bootleg silicone, allegedly acquired from shipments made to the small group of authorized physicians, was being used extensively by plastic surgeons to repair skin defects or simply to provide a filler for wrinkles or furrows. During the same period as the clinical trial, several thousand women in Las Vegas and San Francisco—and a lesser number of men—were injected with silicone fluid, unwitting participants in a parallel, unsupervised "mass experiment" in cosmetic surgery. These individuals received often massive injections of silicone to their body proper to augment breasts or muscle tissue in buttocks and legs. And many of them experienced adverse effects that belied the assertions of nonreactivity and total safety, including development of gangrene that necessitated breast amputation, pain, swelling, and in at least one instance where a breast implant patient was injected with additional silicone, evidence of frank autoimmune disease.

Hindsight

While Dow Corning was assuring the FDA about the non-reactivity of its silicone, several studies were already under way or published that should have cast doubt on the FDA decision. Some reports suggested that inflammatory problems stemming from silicone injections could be serious and should be anticipated before any large-scale undertaking was begun.[9] Dow

Corning arbitrarily dismissed these serious findings as due to contaminants of their fluid. But animal data made available to Dow Corning by 1970 had shown similar chronic inflammatory changes in dogs that had received miniature silicone breast implants some two years earlier. This adverse data was hidden from the medical community and the FDA by Dow Corning, which published only the six-month data in a 1973 medical journal.[10] The full report surfaced only some eighteen years later, during deliberations over the safety of silicone gel breast implants mandated by the FDA. (I originally uncovered this discrepancy in 1984 during a trial where Dow Corning was found guilty of fraud, but the court record was sealed under a protective order lifted in 1991.)

Things were not good on the production front, either. By 1972, two officers of the Dow Corning corporation had been indicted for shipping fifty-five-gallon drums of silicone oil across state lines, in clear violation of the FDA requirement that no more than 50 cc be shipped. A year later, both pleaded nolo contendere. How these questionable uses emerged, and how the plastic surgery community misused this product for treating real and imagined skin problems, is a saga of false hopes, misrepresentation, and vanity.

Dying for Beauty

By 1973, three years after Dow Corning hid its data about chronic inflammatory changes, the first deaths were being reported from injections of silicone. While Dow Corning asserted that these fatalities were the result of illicit use of adulterated silicone, at least one death reported in the *Journal of the American Medical Association* in 1975 was apparently due to "pure" silicone fluid supplied by one of the (unnamed) authorized surgeons of the first Dow Corning protocol.[11] One of the most grisly reports came in the transcript of a phone call I found in FDA files, dated April 5, 1973, from a senior toxicologist at the Georgia Crime Lab in Atlanta to Dow Corning, concerning a Macon, Georgia, woman who had been injected in her breast with silicone fluid. She died apparently right after receiving the illicit injection in her breasts from a pharmaceutical salesman. Her autopsy report showed extensive emboli of silicone in her brain and lungs, any one of which could have compromised her blood circulation and killed her.

In 1975, even as these ominous communications were being received by the FDA, Dow Corning filed a New Drug Application for formal approval of silicone oil as a drug but withdrew it a scant year later at the behest of FDA officials. In its September 14, 1976, letter, the FDA noted Dow Corning's "inability to control misuses of [the] product." Whatever misgivings the FDA might have had at this time about safety (and there were many) were submerged in the polite legalese of the letter.

In spite of this setback, in December 1976 Dow Corning amended its NDA and asked for its further review. This time, the protocol would be strictly limited to treating severe facial deformities; there would be an assigned "independent" medical monitor; and Dow Corning would limit all work to five years. Astonishingly, in view of the spate of adverse reports, this new, more limited NDA was approved, and still more women with facial defects were injected on a "compassionate use" basis. While many of this new group of women benefited in the short run, others (like a young nurse in Salt Lake City who had received a series of over forty injections to her face) had disastrous results. In her case (which I reviewed as an expert witness for the plaintiff), tissue reactions to the silicone had destroyed much of her remaining facial tissue, requiring dozens of additional cosmetic surgeries that left her disfigured and in constant pain. She sued Dow Corning and her doctor. Both settled out of court.

Aftermath

At the end of both programs in the late 1970s, a statistical review by the Biometric Research Institute criticized all of the Dow Corning studies as being "nonblinded" throughout, meaning that both patient and investigator knew when and where the silicone was being injected. There were no control injections. In the opinion of the review team, this single fact was the greatest flaw of the experiment, since it undermined the likelihood of independent and objective judgment of the outcome of the work. Considering that the primary purpose of the study was to establish the long-term safety of silicone, it is remarkable that of 709 of the original dermatologists' patients followed, 487 were lost to follow-up and their data irretrievably lost.

Whether or not this was an indication of untrammeled success (no follow-up was needed, some claimed) or embarrassment over poor outcome is anyone's guess. In some surgeons' hands, as we saw with Dr. Orentreich, 10 percent of the patients had less than desired outcomes. And an indeterminate number of additional patients had such poor outcomes that they ended up successfully suing Dow Corning for providing the untested product in the first place.

Illicit use of silicone continued during the 1980s, culminating in a report from France in 1983 of a near disastrous complication following silicone injections: pneumonitis. This sometimes fatal inflammation of the lungs developed in three transsexual males injected subcutaneously with silicone,[12] suggesting that distant migration of the material could produce serious organ damage.

Caveat Emptor

As late as June of 1991, while I was in attendance in Congress as a speaker at a congressional hearing headed by Ted Weiss, the late representative from New York, a physician informed the FDA that he was continuing to use silicone injections to treat women with cosmetic problems. While he was upbraided for his brazen actions in violation of FDA authority, no plastic surgeon who has used silicone has been formally charged or prosecuted then or now by the federal government. Anecdotal reports suggest that silicone injections are still being done in the privacy of plastic surgeon offices in Southern California, and direct augmentation of the lips with silicone in Mexican clinics is being openly advertised on the Spanish-speaking cable station in our area. And while silicone is broadly outlawed, plastic surgeons still apply a technique with dangers of its own, replacing thinned subcutaneous fat with direct injections of the patient's own body fat.

The use of "contained" silicone in the form of implants is itself the subject of intense litigation. Over 440,000 women have filed suit as part of a class action against major manufacturers. While the controversy still rages over just how sick these women may be and if certain diseases are in fact overrepresented among silicone breast implant recipients (two recent studies suggest they are not), the FDA has taken a prudent course. In 1992, it suspended all but experimental use of silicone gel implants for cosmetic purposes, while permitting their more general use for reconstruction surgery after operations for breast cancer. In 1995, Dow Corning filed for bankruptcy.

Comment

For some, such as Dr. Marcia Agell, senior editor of the *New England Journal of Medicine*, the prior free availability of silicone breast implants was warranted by a justified willingness of women to take risks with their own bodies. I have no problem with this view, as long as recipients are informed of the dangers and benefits. But until 1991, no implant manufacturer's package inserts adequately disclosed the full panoply of dangers associated with silicone. As a result, for the countless women (and men) who undertook their cosmetic risks out of shame, fear of social ostracism, or self-loathing and the others who paid the price in health impairment, the concept of "free choice" rings hollow. In no other field of medicine is "choice" so inextricably mixed with psychological and social forces. What passes for free choice elsewhere may be coercion in the plastic surgeon's office. And the full disclosure of the risks for such procedures began to represent the full truth only after 1992, when the FDA undertook to supervise clinical trials of silicone-based breast implants.

If we have learned anything from the silicone story, it is that our cultural obsession with beauty can blind us to our own inevitable biological limitations. Our quest for beauty nonetheless continues to fuel a multibillion-dollar industry in cosmetic products.

ELEVEN

Cosmetology

The adornment and beautification of the skin is a fundamental cultural need. Cultural artifacts from prehistoric and more recent epochs attest to the amount of human energy invested in developing colorants, tattooing devices, and ornaments to augment the attractiveness of the human form. The recently uncovered five-thousand-year-old body of the Ice Age Man in the Italian Alps provides one of the only mirrors into this behavior in our distant past: his entire upper torso was tattooed. Virtually every preliterate culture (and many of the literate ones) developed an extraordinary array of skin treatments to amplify facial and bodily features, from the tremendous lip-expanding disks of the Ubangis in Africa to the tusk-piercing practices of New Guinean natives. In other cultures, the adornments were more superficial and transient.

Cosmetics were actually made in the temples of ancient Egypt, as writings from the time of Ptolemy III (237 B.C.) attest. Ancient Egyptians were renowned for their unguents, oils, and cosmetics, especially for those designed to highlight the eyes. One particular eye makeup called kohl was the modern-day precursor of eye shadow. Following the collapse of the Roman

Empire, cosmetic use declined and a pure white complexion prevailed as the norm of beauty. In the Middle Ages, arsenic was used to heighten the complexion and white lead powder to tint the skin and dye the hair, both with toxic results to an untold number of aficionados. But thereafter, colorants came back into favor, with intense purples, browns, and shades of green for eye shadow and red predominating for rouge, especially among prostitutes. In Elizabethan times, Englishwomen rouged their cheeks and painted their lips in vermilion hues, while maintaining a stark white contrast for their facial makeup. Thus throughout historical times, the desire for coloration and adornments ensured a widespread, cross-cultural use of both natural and artificial cosmetics.

The most plausible reason for this universal behavior is evident to any biologist steeped in evolutionary theory: almost alone in the animal kingdom, the external human form has evolved devoid of colorful ornamentation. Sexual selection in other animals, particularly birds, has led to the development of often extraordinary accouterments to augment the attractiveness of one sex (usually male) to the other. Charles Darwin was the first to posit that the remarkable achievement of peacock tail eyespots and vivid baboon facial markings have a common evolutionary origin: sexual selection.

Should the one sex (usually the female) elect a partner with particular distinguishing characteristics that have a genetic basis, those features will be amplified and selected over time. The male that drew the largest number of females to his harem perpetuated the largest portion of his genes. Often in the wild, females are observed to select males with particularly symmetrical features. As a compensation for this investment in symmetrical beauty, contemporary evolutionists posit that males laden with as many adornments as the peacock had to have an extra measure of vitality and genetic "stamina": hence, the perpetuation of often extreme sexually selected characters like the peacocks' or bowerbirds' tails may actually enhance the species' overall fitness.

In humans, sexual selection has probably accounted for many of the racial features that characterize relatively isolated populations, including differences in skin coloration, facial features, and hair color. These features pale before the more florid natural cosmetic ornamentation that characterize our nearest primate ancestors. The exuberant purple, red, and blue coloration of dominant male baboon faces or the reddened and swollen flesh of the genital areas of female chimpanzees in heat exemplify the extremes of natural selection.

A reasonable question for an evolutionary anthropologist to ask is why, with the notable exception of the accumulation of fat stores in the buttocks known as steatopygia, similarly graphic features have not evolved in humans. The answer appears to be embedded in the diversity of adornments possible through cultural evolution. Absent the natural enhancement of beauty that sexual selection in the wild promotes, the human species has relied on decoration, enhancement, or concealment to augment the attractiveness of our superficial features. The consequence of this evolutionary void for humans is that cultural evolution has supplanted the need for physical evolution. Facial pigments, lipstick, eye shadow, tattoos, and blush provide the sexual cues otherwise relegated to natural or sexual selection.

Tattooing

Being the most visible manifestation of our individuality, the skin evolved radically over time as a marker of tribal affinity, race, and cultural groups. With the advent of culture, artificial coloring, tattooing, and other ornamental distortions of the skin became a mainstay. Such tattooing capitalized on the fact that injections or scarifications that just penetrated the uppermost layer of the skin could deposit materials like charcoal, sepia ink, or pigments into the upper dermis, where they would remain relatively stable over time. The apotheosis of tattooing as a cultural icon was probably reached with the New Zealand Maori, who used extensive body and facial tattooing to identify tribal origins and to accentuate the fierceness of their warriors. When done with scrupulous hygienic care, the process of tattooing is itself relatively innocuous, aside from the initial pain, which can be considerable. However, a little-appreciated side effect is the development of psoriasis in the tattooed area. This reaction is known to dermatologists as Koebner's phenomenon and reflects the predilection of psoriasis to traumatized skin areas.

Providing the amenities that permit such adornments is today the province of an entire industry of cosmetics. Medical advancements have radically extended the range of cosmetic interventions, including enhancement of secondary sexual characteristics, notably the breast, buttocks, and lips. But the largest amount of energy has gone to refining and modifying the skin.

Preoccupation with Skin Beauty

Surveys show that we think about our skin more than any other part of our anatomy. Our spending habits show this: depending on our age and social class, Americans spend 6–10 percent of their expendable income on cosmetic products. Teenagers may double this proportion. This expenditure is also a reflection of how much we invest emotionally in our outward appearance. Cosmetic companies ensure that we put little faith in natural beauty. Through extensive advertising, they "encourage" us to pay attention to pores that are too large; noses that are misshapen or at least too shiny; skin blemishes; lips that are too thin and undercolored; and skin that is too oily, too dry, or too pale or dark. Cosmetic firms play on our vanity and vulnerability to societal expectations. They promote moisturizers and lotions that promise to do away with complexion problems and hide horrid brown spots.

But sometimes this treatment can be counterproductive. Many of the most heavily promoted products seal in oils that make acne worse or accentuate dryness by stripping away skin layers or oils that normally protect the skin from dehydration. At an extreme, some products may do harm elsewhere while being concentrated on the skin. Examples include the genotoxic chemical hydroquinone, which is used to "correct" liver spots; isotretinoin or Accutane for treating cystic acne (discussed in chapter 6); and some of the chemical peels designed to cause exfoliation of facial skin.

Less visibly, many lotions or emollients may silently permit the ingress of hazardous chemicals by encouraging their permeation through the skin. Harsh chemicals can dissolve essential body oils and even defat the skin. Others, like the para-aminobenzoic acid (PABA) in sunscreens, are highly allergenic. A whole new group of cosmetic companies like Garden Botanika and the Body Shop have emerged that promise "safe" and natural products with fewer of these side effects. They emphasize some traditional skin treatments that have not yet seen a full-blown resurgence. One of these was known to the ancients. Sheep skin contains ample amounts of lanolin, a natural waterproofing agent and protectant. Sheep shearers are renowned for the softness of their hands and are rumored to roll naked on their shearing tables after work just to ensure that the rest of their body receives similar exposure.

Drying Out

As already mentioned, cosmetic companies play on our atavistic anxiety about dehydration, the deep-rooted fear that left unprotected and exposed to the elements, we would dry out and wither away. They promote soaps and moisturizers "guaranteed" to keep our skin hydrated and young. But many cosmetic products, especially soaps and skin "tighteners," do the opposite, accelerating drying and promoting the appearance of aged skin by removing the natural oils that protect the skin's surface. Exfoliation can do the same thing, by providing a speedy way to accelerate the natural loss of surface skin. By revealing the more vital tissue just under the surface, a clay masque or "chemical peel" will provide a transient appearance of more youthful skin. Occasionally, through errors in formulation or ultrasensitivity in the client, a chemical peel can be extraordinarily harmful, literally burning the skin. The Japanese err on the side of safety and use rice hulls to abrade the skin for the same effect. But in time, repeated bouts of exfoliation will exhaust and desiccate the skin, as the treatment overtakes the skin's natural ability for self-restoration.

Natural Skin

Every so often, the fashion industry recognizes that beauty is just skin deep. Few natural features are more alluring than are uncovered lips and fresh, dewy skin. The "natural" look stays around for a while, but so few models can sustain a relaxed, untrammeled skin that the trend dies out almost as soon as it begins. As every designer knows, cosmetic products produce "cover girls" by covering.

This unwillingness to leave well enough alone extends to the medical profession as well. Topical antibiotics like cleomycin that can act only on a few follicles or systemic ones like tetracycline that concentrate in the skin but do virtually nothing to eliminate entrenched bacteria are prescribed with abandon for teenagers with common acne. Antifungal medications now available over the counter probably do as much to encourage the outgrowth of resistant organisms and irritate the skin as they do to heal it. And the popularity of vaginal douches with antiyeast medications obscures the likelihood that most of the yeast overgrowth is due to bacterial suppression with antibiotics in the first place.[1]

While every medical school has a department of dermatology, few schools teach natural healing as a form of skin care. Left to its own devices and kept out of the sun, our skin is a marvelous organ that ensures our survival under extremes of dryness or heat. Because of an elegantly simple system that maintains its bacteria-inhibiting acidity through secretion of sebum, sweat, and salts and dampens its outer layers continuously, the skin rarely if ever needs the lubrication and "moisture" added by cosmetics. And under duress and abrasion, the skin readily "sheds" significant numbers of dead cells as a kind of buffer against deeper damage. This shedding takes with it unwanted fungal and yeast cells and keeps the skin replenished with healthy cells and their by-products. With continued wear or pressure, the skin adapts and strengthens itself, adding thickened keratin layers where needed. In an earlier time, the calluses on hands and feet so zealously buffed away by the pumice stones of manicurists were once admired as signs of strength and essential adaptations critical to barefoot survival.

Beauty Is Skin Deep

Smooth and supple skin is the epitome of beauty. As California fashion photographer Ron Bolander recently said to me, in his industry "skin is everything." With age, skin dries out and loses its elasticity and wrinkles become the norm. Anything and everything to retard this inevitable transformation has been tried over history. In ancient Syria, the lung of a camel was laid on the skin "for a complexion like wax." The ancient Egyptians used hippopotamus fat, gazelle dung, and ground donkey teeth mixed with honey along with writing fluid to keep the skin young. In Rome, women maintained their youthful appearance by treating their faces with a paste made of honey, wine sediment, and finely ground narcissus bulbs. Henry III slept in a night mask of flour and egg whites. And in the seventeenth century, women slept with their faces covered in a mask of silk or leather stretched to the fullest to "erase" aging lines.[2]

The biological basis for these remedies is often obscure, but at least some, like the Egyptian preparation containing writing fluid and honey, were likely to have proven beneficial. Natural inks are rich in tannins, which have great antibacterial activity, and honey, by virtue of its high sugar concentration, also inhibits bacterial growth. Both could have helped the complexion.

Modern-day treatments have included derivatives of vitamin A, embryo extracts, and exotic creams containing vegetable secretions like aloe and derivatives of other plants from cucumbers to rosemary. Too much of any one of these applications—especially vitamin A derivatives like Retin-A—can of course be harmful.

Then as today, beauty was often a trade-off between short-term appearance and long-term harm.

The Cult of Youthfulness

In the end, all beautification treatments have a common core: they are all attempts to keep the skin young. To understand something of how cosmetics approach this elusive goal, we must understand the basics of skin biology. In youth, virtually all skin has a natural suppleness and smoothness. Its pH is naturally low (around 5.6), but not so low as to lead to denaturation of skin proteins. To maintain these features, it is essential to have sufficient water absorbed by the cells in the outermost layers of the skin, the stratum corneum. When the stratum corneum loses water, it stiffens, sloughs, and becomes hard and even brittle.

Maintaining good hydration, the water-carrying capacity of the skin, is the sine qua non of good cosmetic practice. In spite of intensive advertisements to the contrary, the water carried in the skin can be "added" only partially from the outside. Most of the water is furnished through the aqueous portion of the blood known as plasma, which seeps through interstices between the lipid layers in the epidermal barrier. As we saw in chapter 4, slightly salty water constantly percolates upward to the skin surface through the underlying dermis, much as a plant receives replenishment from its roots. Normally, most of this water is retained at or near the skin surface by an insulating, microscopic layer of natural lipids that are produced from the sebaceous glands and the keratin-producing cells themselves.

Evaporation of this water may be aggravated by climate extremes, as anyone who has gone outside on a dry, blustery winter day knows. The more extreme forms of desiccation like chapped lips or cracked skin are usually the result of unprotected exposure to severe weather conditions that disrupt the lipid layer and abrade the overlying epidermis. Exposure to solvents in the workplace or to household products such as dishwashing liquids can rapidly accomplish the same end, drying the skin unnaturally and making it vulnerable to eczema or other skin disorders. In extreme circumstances, such as during repetitive solvent exposure to workers from dipping machine parts into degreasing agents, the deeper layers of the skin can be defatted, leading to thin, excoriated, and damaged skin that cracks and loses its natural elasticity and suppleness.

Preserving or restoring this first line of defense through improved lubrication at the skin surface, protection of the lipid layer, and conservation of the water contained at the skin surface is the first line of business in any successful occupational hygiene program or cosmetic dermatology practice. Oils, Vaseline, and emollients, however, do not so much lubricate as they seal in the skin's natural moisture under a vapor barrier. (It is critical to avoid trapping bacteria under such impermeable barriers, since they may inadvertently provide a nutrient bath for a suppurating infection.)

Once this first principle of water conservation is recognized, maintaining a hydrated and water-repellent skin surface is seemingly straightforward: avoid excessive exposure to drying agents, especially harsh soaps, detergents, and solvents. When in dry climates or dehumidified spaces—especially on airplanes or in air-conditioned rooms—use of periodic wet packs can restore some water lost through evaporation at the skin surface.

When washing the skin, using cool water and little soap can improve skin quality. And when lost through age or exposure, lipids can be restored through judicious use of skin creams *when the skin is still wet.* This last suggestion is a secret well known to cosmetologists but lost on many people who apply cold cream only after a vigorous scrubbing and dehydrating wash coupled with a brisk toweling-off.

Adverse Reactions

But achieving these ends without producing damaging secondary effects is an art form in itself. Creams with a solid foundation of compatible lipids like those found in avocado are useful in keeping skin supple. Lotions generally contain fewer lipids than do creams. As a result, they are less likely to restore this critical skin component. Some risks are involved in the overuse of hand creams, including exacerbation of psoriasis, entrapment of bacteria, and fungal overgrowth.

A widely respected dermatology textbook argues convincingly for the limited use of some products to replace lost lipids with minimal side effects.[3] Potentially toxic products that restore water to seriously dried skin are usually available by prescription only. Ironically, the "secret" ingredients in these products are substances that by themselves are caustic or aesthetically objectionable, such as urea and lactic acid. These chemicals are added to ensure that a greater amount of water is held in the cream and made available to the skin. If you have breaks in the skin, these ingredients will probably sting and irritate. The addition of bath oils, a time-honored tradition, actually provides little by way of lipid replacement and is generally a waste of time.

Irritated Skin

As we saw in chapter 6, when skin is inflamed or irritated, or rashes have developed as a result of exposure to an external irritant or allergen, dermatologists routinely prescribe corticosteroids to restore the skin to its normal appearance. When these often potent medicines were first introduced in the 1950s they received such instant notoriety that they have formed the mainstay of skin treatments ever since. In spite of the fact that extensive use can lead to serious side effects, many low-concentration (0.5 to 1.0 percent) corticosteroid creams can now be purchased over the counter.

This ready accessibility should not lull the consumer into a state of complacency. The same anti-inflammatory properties of skin creams with corticosteroids can actually suppress the immune system if large surface areas of the body are exposed. As discussed in chapter 8, with widespread application in a child with extensive poison ivy or oak—and especially if an occlusive dressing is used to keep the steroid in contact with the skin longer—a generalized depression of the immune system is possible.[4]

These steroid-containing creams are sometimes used to treat acne, an inflammation surrounding a sebaceous gland that is usually accompanied by a low-level bacterial infection. Typical low-potency corticosteroids containing hydrocortisone can suppress this inflammation but do little to deal with the underlying causes of acneform eruptions, which are usually a combination of dietary and hormonal factors.

Testing for Safety

🖎 Cosmetics generally have to pass muster with the FDA as "hypoallergenic" and nonirritating. In the recent past, the cosmetics industry relied on dubious and overly simplistic means to establish these properties. Ointments, creams, oils, and soaps were all tested for irritancy in what was known as the "Draize test," a procedure in which the test chemical was intentionally placed into the eyes of unanesthetized rabbits to reveal any inflammatory properties. Short-term (thirty days and less) toxicity testing sufficed to clear a cosmetic product as biocompatible. And allergenicity was evaluated by "patch testing" human volunteers.

As a health official, I evaluated one such program in the late 1970s. In 1977, I visited the notorious Vacaville Prison in California, where the most violent and recidivist prisoners in the state are housed (including Charles Manson). I was astonished to find hardened prisoners "volunteering" to have dozens of patches of lipsticks and facial creams put on their shaved backs. At any other place, volunteers wearing cosmetics this way would be the butt of jokes or even receive outright abuse. Here, a cosmetic patch was considered a badge of courage and a rare contact with the outside world.

Even after such rigorous testing, many cosmetic products still produce florid skin reactions in sensitive individuals, perhaps because a teenager's face bears scant resemblance to a convict's back. This is especially true of sunscreens, antiperspirants, and deodorant soaps. All three of these products are designed to contain active ingredients that bind to skin proteins to produce their desired effects. Human variation in sensitivity ensures that even after the most intensive testing, many cosmetics like these will still be allergenic to some consumers.[5]

Today, numerous cosmetic companies are moving toward testing that is "animal free." At a local mall, cosmetic salespeople wear T-shirts that declare "No Animal Testing." This means that neither Draize testing nor patch testing is being done. While I believe that the Draize test is unusually cruel, there is no substitute for *some* noninvasive animal testing (such as patch tests) to ensure safety. The only alternative is for the consumer be the guinea pig or to devise sensitive tissue culture assays to measure the same properties.

Wrinkling with Old Age

One pervasive myth about skin is that wrinkling and loss of elasticity are an inevitable consequence of aging. In fact, individuals who spend little or no time in the sun show remarkably young-looking skin well into their seventies. An old friend, Joe Cavanna of Blue Canyon, California, lived in the back room of a bar in one of the harshest environments in the Sierra Nevada mountains, yet his skin was as young and supple as a baby's. Joe's secret: He never left the bar!

Sunlight, and possibly the presence of harsh chemicals in cigarette smoke, cause much damage to the underlying layers of the skin and inevitably produce visible damage after years of exposure. But evidence of solar damage accrues slowly, perhaps explaining our continuing indulgence in sunbathing. And a tan affords no permanent protection for these chronic effects. After about thirty years of relatively constant exposure to the sun, even the most heavily tanned person will show characteristic skin changes. This includes thinning, drying, and loss of elasticity.

While the wrinkling associated with solar exposure is indistinguishable from that produced by the passage of time, the effect of sunlight is to accelerate these changes and make them more pronounced. Natural skin lines, the signs of "character" that result from the repetitive use of certain muscle groups, are often greatly accentuated after protracted sunlight. Frown and smile lines alike are thrown in stark relief in the sun- and weather-etched face. Elsewhere, particularly on the back of the neck, the skin takes on a leathery and folded appearance with chronic solar exposure.

With continued intense exposure to sunlight into late middle age, lakes of blood may collect on the lips and ears, and lines of tiny blood vessels may appear on the cheeks. Sometimes an otherwise mysterious pattern of small yellow papules appear on the cheeks or forehead or yellowish nodules may arise on the back of the neck and around the eyes. Circular areas on the exposed dorsum of the hand may become scaly and begin to form raised, scaly papules called keratoses. These lesions, also known as senile keratoses, are often precancerous and may lead to squamous cell carcinomas. In all, the effects of sunlight clearly accelerate the normal changes in the skin that accompany aging. Although skin may thin and become less resilient with age in any person, sun or no sun, the proliferation of wrinkles so commonly associated with illustrations of characters out of the Wild West is a concomitant of the wear and tear of sun and weather—and not aging per se.

Solar skin damage goes down below the epidermal layer to damage the very "soul" of the skin, the elastic fibers and collagen that make up the dermis itself and give skin its firm, resilient feel. A simple test of your "age factor" is to take a pinch of skin in two fingers on the back of your hand. Lift gently until it forms a small tent and then let it go. The speed with which the skin snaps back (or sags) into place, flat on the surface of your hand, is a direct reflection of the remaining elasticity of these fibers.

If you have been outdoors for a large part of your adult life, there is a good chance that your hands have been exposed to significant amounts of sunlight. If that is so, your "rebound" age may actually be older than your biological age, for sunlight causes a high rate of damage to the collagen and other dermal proteins. Young skin retains its elasticity. Until the age of forty-five, the skin still normally rebounds in two seconds or less. By the age of sixty-five, the rebound rate can be as long as twenty seconds. Just five years later, it will sag slowly, taking up to fifty seconds to return to its original surface. Where skin has been damaged from too much sunlight, longer retraction times can show up even in "young" skin.

While still too imprecise to serve as a scientific biomarker of aging, this dramatic loss of elasticity is clearly telling us something about changes in the skin—and, indirectly, about the way we age as a whole.

Wrinkles?

For cosmetologists, the $64,000 question is whether or not such natural effects can be thwarted or—better still—reversed. Most facial wrinkles, especially those in the chin and neck, result from the habitual pull of muscles that lie parallel to the stretch lines of the skin. Elsewhere, around the mouth and eyes, wrinkles form from the constant action of muscles that run perpendicular to the stress lines. The puckered appearance of the mouth and crow's-feet of the eyes mark the areas where skin lies over the orbicularis or circular muscles that control the contour of these regions. Wrinkles that take on a crisscross appearance have no specific cause. These wrinkles may simply be contracture lines and resemble the random "cracking" of a brittle surface, much as a dry lake will form cracks and fissures as the once-moist mud and clay contracts.

The critical function of the dermis in such age marks has not been lost on the cosmetic pharmaceutical industry. Each year, literally thousands of new products are tested to provide better skin protection or appearance. Of all these "new" cosmetics, it is remarkable that the most effective are those that directly influence the dermal-epidermal relationship. Skin creams or masks that seek to control wrinkles by "ironing" them out inevitably fail because of the repetitive stresses that regenerate wrinkle lines and because of the elastic memory in the underlying fibers that bring them back to their original shape after deformation.

Two views prevail about the significance (or lack thereof) of wrinkling. One, championed by gerontologist Leonard Hayflick, is that wrinkles are incidental to health. According to Hayflick, "Wrinkled skin is not unhealthy skin."[6] If we think otherwise, it is the result of our cultural conditioning rather than any biological truth. For Hayflick, our negative attitudes about wrinkling are pure fluff, something we are taught. The apotheosis of the Hayflick view is captured by Albert Kligman, a University of Pennsylvania dermatologist. Kligman is quoted as stating that "it is not clear why one should bother to study cutaneous aging. After all, no one dies of old skin!"[7]

It is true that a tremendous amount of advertising is directed toward our preference for smooth skin. But is it simply aesthetics that drives the demand for youthful appearance? Hayflick's view is that aged skin is "not clinically significant."[8] I disagree. As Hayflick himself points out, two-thirds of people over the age of seventy have skin conditions that warrant a trip to the doctor. While it is true that no one dies directly of "skin failure," many fall ill and die from diseases like scleroderma and invasive squamous cell carcinoma, both of which are correlated with age-linked changes in the skin. (In scleroderma, collagen ages prematurely under autoimmune attack, while squamous cell carcinoma shows the statistical characteristics of an age-associated cancer.)

Much research shows the importance of an intact and robust underlayment for the health of the skin. When the dermis is damaged or thinned by age, the epidermis is not as vital, and its blood supply may be compromised. As mentioned in the section on skin cancer in chapter 6, there are even biologists who believe the fundamental basis for skin cancer arising in the skin is a damaged (including solar-damaged) dermis and *not* a direct effect of sunlight on the overlying skin itself. While the primary villain in producing skin damage is the sun, other factors can contribute to premature aging of the skin.

Wrinkling and Cigarette Smoking

Over time, of course, we all will age and crinkle up—especially at those stress lines where the face has been subjected to repeated stretching and folding. A common myth is that exaggeration of these features occurs through typical facial responses to the elements like squinting and grimacing. The Marlboro Man, that enduring American symbol of virility, is always shown lighting up in the great outdoors, his wrinkled visage scrunched up as he leans over to shield his smoke from the wind. With such powerful images, it is understandable how this "wear and tear" myth of character lines evolved. Cigarette manufacturers encouraged this interpretation by using visual images to stress that while the extreme lifestyle of a cowhand might lead to a wrinkled countenance, continuous exposure to the elements was the explanation, not smoking.

A few long-term dermatology researchers were not to be deterred by this subtle propaganda, believing that smokers are more prone to develop wrinkles over time than are nonsmokers. For most researchers, the putative association still did not make sense: how could smoke cause wrinkles? How could a substance that is inhaled into the lungs affect the skin? Many investigators simply assumed it was the Marlboro Man effect: people who smoked were just more likely to work or play outdoors. Indeed, until 1995, most researchers accepted the coincidental association between cigarettes and wrinkling, believing that solar damage explained all there was to know about aged skin.

The issue rested there until a team of researchers at the Kaiser Permanente Medical Care Program in Oakland, California, and the University of California at San Francisco performed a meticulous comparison of 228 smokers, 456 former smokers, and 227 nonsmokers. Participants were asked to leave all smoking paraphernalia at home and not to reveal their smoking habits to a review team who were to observe the number, depth, and frequency of facial wrinkles.[9] (Ironically, the study was supported by funds that were provided by taxes generated by smokers through the Tobacco Surtax Fund of the State of California.) Solar exposure was matched in all groups.

The results were dramatic. In both men and women forty years and older, the number of cigarettes a person smoked correlated *directly* with the extent of their facial wrinkles. Women and men cigarette smokers were two to three times as likely to have moderate to severe wrinkling compared with nonsmokers. According to the research team, this apparent dose-response relationship can be explained at least three ways. First, something in cigarette smoke directly damages the skin. Since cigarette smoke is known to damage collagen and elastin in the lungs, the research team reasoned, systemically absorbed smoke might cause the facial damage. Alternately, perhaps smoke blown across the face produces a direct drying or irritation of the skin. A third way cigarette smoke can damage the skin is to constrict the arterioles that provide blood to its surface. Another research team suggested a fourth way—that smoking causes wrinkling indirectly by reducing the amount of vitamin A the body is able to absorb. The resulting loss of this essential antioxidant may diminish the body's level of protection against oxygen radicals known to damage DNA and connective tissue.[10]

But a fifth explanation is possible. What if cigarette smoke causes aging changes throughout the body, including damage not only to collagen and elastin molecules, but actual genetic damage to body cells generally? Might not the aging-related changes seen in the skin be akin to the clonal damage that cigarette smoke derivatives like benzoapyrene (a major cigarette smoke contaminant) produce in other target organs like the cells that line the blood vessels in the heart? If DNA damage leads to proliferation of prematurely aged, precancerous clones of damaged cells, cigarette smoke might cause an irrevocable aging effect. One test of this idea is to determine if cigarette smoking contributes to skin cancer irrespective of exposure to sunlight, an idea that is as yet untested.

Retarding Aging in the Skin

Over the last few decades, only a handful of products have proven capable of maintaining youthful-appearing skin. Among the most potent of these are those that either replace or "rejuvenate" the collagen in the dermis. In fact, so powerful is the presence of youthful, springy collagen molecules that whole companies have sprung up that sell collagen derivatives to the plastic surgery community for injection into sun-damaged or wrinkled skin. So-called collagen injections are not without risk, however. Should the body recognize the collagen (most often made from specially treated cow collagen) as foreign, the ensuing immune reaction can wreak havoc throughout the body's other collagen stores. A mixed connective tissue disease in which collagen is attacked throughout the body can result.

A better approach appears to be the use of the natural vitamins that keep the skin youthful appearing. These include vitamin E or A and its derivative, known as the retinoids. Retin-A, or tretinoin, is one such derivative. When placed on the skin in suitable concentrations, Retin-A creams can produce an artificial stimulation of the basal skin layer, which produces the epidermis. A subsequent thickening of this layer can often obscure wrinkles and give the skin a more youthful appearance. Another theory is that Retin-A can encourage the regeneration of lost and damaged collagen in the dermis. New research shows that over time, repetitive use of Retin-A can lead to replacement of collagen and repair of minor degenerative changes in the skin, as long as no further solar damage is permitted. Solar exposure of Retin-A–treated skin can exaggerate the minor inflammatory changes that sometimes accompany therapy, negating any beneficial effects. A major concern is that Retin-A's major side effects will only belatedly be known, since its use as an antiaging cream has only recently been FDA approved. The same is true for new skin creams that deliver controlled amounts of antioxidants to the underlying skin.

In the end, aging of the skin is as inevitable as taxes. The best we may do to stave off this decline is to acknowledge one key fact: Sunlight is the skin's nemesis.

TWELVE

The UV Story

The ability of sunlight to age the skin prematurely has been recognized for at least two hundred years and in folklore for much longer. But the full role of the sun in damaging the skin's regenerative and protective roles has been recognized only in the last two decades. In spite of this awareness, the medical establishment itself has encouraged solar overindulgence.

Sunlight as Therapy

Western medicine's infatuation with sunlight as a panacea began in the darkness of the Industrial Revolution. With the invention of the sanitarium in the mid-1800s in tuberculosis-ravaged Europe, full exposure to the sun became the treatment of choice for consumption. At sanitaria throughout the Alps of Italy, Germany, and Austria, tuberculosis patients were prescribed up to eight hours or more of full exposure to the highly energized, actinic rays of the mountain sun as "therapy" for their chronic and debilitating state. In the pristine environs above the diseased lowlands, health was equated with a ruddy, tanned complexion. As later captured in Thomas Mann's novel *The Magic Mountain*, the sunlight-filled rooms of the mountain sanitarium became a world unto itself, where the thermometer measured the passage of time, and days were passed in repose under the beneficient rays of the sun.

In 1900, inspired by this illusory equation of solar exposure and perfect health, Danish dermatologist Niels Finsen invented an electric lamp that could mimic the full spectrum light of the sun. Like many other physicians of his day, Finsen believed that sunlight had curative powers for TB. Among the patients he treated with this artificial sunlight were many infected with the cutaneous form of tuberculosis known as lupus vulgaris. Lupus vulgaris typically caused a horribly disfiguring, exuberant overgrowth of skin on the face, often transforming the nose and surrounding tissues into a distorted red mass. At the Third International Congress of Dermatology in Paris, in a dramatic display of his work, Finsen showed the participants "before" and "after" pictures of patients whom he had "cured" with his new lamp. His audience was astonished. Lupus vulgaris had never before been eradicated. His light therapy spawned an entire new field of medicine known as heliotherapy. Therapy with sunlight was so highly regarded that in 1903 Finsen was awarded the Nobel Prize for his discovery of the sunlamp.

With hindsight, we now know that Finsen's apparent success in treating cutaneous tuberculosis was probably due to the powerful immune-suppressing and anti-inflammatory effects of intense sunlight. The overgrowths of skin tissue in lupus are part of the body's ineffective proliferative reaction to TB, and suppression of this tissue was accomplished by the selective immune cell–killing effects of sunlight. In reality, it is extremely unlikely that Finsen truly "cured" any of his patients of their TB so much as he helped abate their symptoms.

The Promotion of Sunlight

The literary themes that emerged in the 1920s perpetuated this belief in the benefits of sunlight. F. Scott Fitzgerald described tanned young swingers as the trendsetters of the Roaring Twenties in his novel *Tender Is the Night*. By the mid-1920s, the deliberate and, some might say, obsessive pursuit of a bronzed complexion truly began in earnest. Fashion designers like Coco Chanel promoted the suntanned look as the epitome of haute couture, and women young and old sought out the sun. Whereas previous cultural norms praised the wan, pallid complexion of the "stay at home" beauty, the new trend was for a tanned look—albeit one that lacked the outdoorsy, pseudomasculine emphasis of some of today's trendy fashion magazines. In 1944, a Miami pharmacist marketed the first suntan oil, a material designed more to keep the skin from drying out than to offer any substantial protection from overexposure.[1] From the 1950s on, the marketing of suntan aids, from oils to creams, encouraged a whole generation to seek out dangerously long exposures to the sun. In the 1990s, we have just begun to reap the consequences of this innocent obsession with the sun in repeated and increasingly common bouts with skin cancer.

Even today, the medical profession prescribes sunlight therapy for "curing" psoriasis and otherwise self-limiting skin conditions like acne. (My own family doctor repeatedly treated my acne with UV light when I was an adolescent.) While solar exposure and controlled sunlamp treatments may have a legitimate place in treating such intractable skin conditions as psoriasis, they are still much overused. As I will show, tanning booths and UV light machines remain dangerous sources of ultraviolet radiation. We may look healthy, but a tan is more a sign of skin damage than benefit.

Many of those who still aspire to the well-tanned look so closely linked to affluence and well-being may be disconcerted to learn that "health and sunlight" is an oxymoron. The most important discovery about the skin in the last decade is that in addition to directly inducing skin cancers, exposure to ultraviolet radiation damages the basic defenses of the skin against local cancer and disease-causing microorganisms. Solar exposure is especially harmful when the wavelengths reaching the skin's surface include the ultraviolet range (in a rainbow, the UV wavelengths of light begin just below the purple light in the visible spectrum).[2] UV light in its most dangerous, short-waved forms (UV-C or -B) is normally substantially blocked by the fast-diminishing ozone layer.

Biology of Sunlight

Now keep in mind that *some* sunlight is essential to well-being. The visible wavelengths of light are critical for making vitamin D and for assuring a balanced circadian rhythm that permits normal hours of wakefulness and sleep. As we saw in the chapter on anatomy, the skin is designed to permit these wavelengths to penetrate deeply, triggering vitamin D synthesis and reaching deep within the skull to the pineal gland to encourage the melatonin release necessary for a normal sleep and wakefulness cycle of about twenty-four hours. But the same transparency to sunlight puts the skin at risk.

The longer wavelengths of UV light known as UV-A oxidize and darken existing melanin within a few minutes of exposure. Generally this is an adaptive response and affords an additional front line of defense against further damage. After exposure to the shorter ultraviolet light wavelengths known as UV-B, the skin develops an erythema, a redness of the skin commonly recognized as sunburn. This initial reddening fades quickly after cessation of exposure. Hidden within this at times painful experiences is a molecular battle for damage control. If exposure has been extensive (say, more than fifteen minutes of direct tropical sunlight), the body responds with a delayed sunburn, which develops within a few hours and, as sufferers know, reaches its peak some ten to twelve hours later, usually in the middle of the night. When this delayed erythema occurs, it heralds substantial skin damage. The result is what we call peeling, where whole sheets of epidermis slough off, perhaps the most unsightly reminder of solar excess.

Following a sunburn, epidermal cells develop shrunken, dead nuclei and are called sunburn cells. The blood vessels open up, causing the burning sensation of sunburned skin; plasma leaves the blood and bloats the tissues (edema); and inflammatory cells migrate to the site of greatest exposure. Production and transfer of new melanin from deep in the dermis to near the epidermal junction occurs about two days after the initial exposure. Even the darkest skin will tan and in time become damaged if solar exposure continues unabated. While short exposures can lead to an adaptive tan and little permanent damage, the greatest UV damage occurs in fair-skinned people who visit the tropics and develop severe sunburn. When such burns occur intermittently over a number of years, the stage is set for cancer.

A "good" suntan peaks in about two to three weeks and will fade rather quickly if further exposure does not intervene. A "bad" sunburn, by comparison, can produce headache, nausea, fever, delirium, and even hypotension or fainting.

While no one knows precisely how much UV light is "bad" for you, it is clear that even a relatively small series of exposures can be carcinogenic in animals. A sequence of enough UV light to produce artificial sunburns three times a week for just thirty weeks is sufficient to produce cancer in most strains of mice. Sometimes even controlled tanning can be hazardous. Adults who indulged in tanning treatments fifteen years ago in their youthful quest to look more attractive now make repeated visits to dermatologists to remove cancerous and precancerous sunlight-induced skin lesions on their faces and bodies.

Tanning Booths

In spite of intensive efforts to marshal support for self-protection from the sun, the quest for the healthy "tanned" look remains a national obsession. This elusive goal has led to the proliferation of artificial light sources that can tan the skin, as well as to cosmetics that will mimic the result without any solar exposure. The rationale for developing artificial tanning salons is simple enough, following the age-old American adage "Find a need and fill it." Unfortunately, the popularity of tanning booths may be putting even more people at risk from sunlight-mediated damage than existed before their invention. The basis for this modern-day "improvement" over the sun is not hard to find.

For many years, it has been assumed that the harmful effects of sunlight are limited to the spectrum of UV radiation concentrated in the B range—that is, 290 to 320 nanometers in wavelength. (Normally UV in the most harmful C range fails to penetrate the atmosphere.) This misconception is critical for the licensing decisions made for tanning booths, in which current regulations limit the use of lamps that have minimal (1 percent or less) UV-B and instead concentrate most of their radiation in the A range, from 320 to 400 nanometers.

With just the UV-A as the dominant wavelength, regulators have been offered assurances that any adverse effects from tanning booths will be "limited" to accelerated aging.[3] Given the fact that UV-A and UV-B radiation work synergistically to tan (and to produce skin cancer), this is more to be hoped for than proven. Of course, sunlight-induced accelerated aging is of concern in and of itself.

That UV light in general actually does cause accelerated aging is no longer a matter of conjecture. After exposure to sunlight, skin cells show a dramatically limited ability to grow in tissue culture compared with their normal life spans. As gerontologist Leonard Hayflick observes, one indication of how much damage sunlight does is to measure the proliferative ability of cells in exposed versus unexposed regions of the body: the cells from the sun-exposed surface of the hand turn out to be much more limited in their proliferative abilities than are those from the armpit.[4]

There is strong suspicion that cancer is not far behind the current tanning fad. Unfortunately, most of the data we have about cancer risks focuses on the few anecdotal reports of individuals who have developed full-blown malignancies after exposure. Most of the hard data on UV and cancer comes from animal studies. But a recent case report strongly suggests what many have long suspected: The concentrated artificial sunlight needed to produce a "good tan" can be cancer provoking, particularly in susceptible or unusually sensitive individuals.

Keeping That Tan

The case in question concerns a red-haired woman from northern England who sought out the "perfect tan" from artificial sunlight.[5] She had virtually no skin-damaging exposure to sunlight as a child. In part, we surmise, her exposure was limited because her mother recognized that with freckled skin and little of the eumelanin (literally "good melanin") needed for tanning, she burned easily if exposed to the sun. Previously she had been abroad only for a two-week period and had never exposed her full body to the sun outdoors. However, beginning in 1982, she underwent twice weekly full-body tanning bed treatments for almost four years. Each time she sunbathed in the nude for approximately thirty minutes, the prescribed time to get a good tan. And tan she did, just enough to keep her coming back.

The tanning parlor used a sunlamp with only minimal (1 percent) UV-B radiation. The patient was not unduly sensitive to UV radiation and had no special genetically based disorders that predisposed her to sunlight-mediated damage. But when at the age of thirty-six she was examined (eight years after her tanning booth exposure), she was found to have developed the following tumors: a wartlike keratoacanthoma on her leg; a basal cell carcinoma on her temple; a squamous cell carcinoma on her chest; and multiple basal cell cancerlike lesions called Bowen's disease on her breasts and buttocks. Most remarkably, this patient had never had any known *natural* sun exposure to these last two areas.

The authors of the study were convinced that her multiple lesions were induced by her tanning booth experience and recommended that no one with an increased risk of skin cancer use such salons. Their list of what they meant by "increased risk" included persons with multiple skin nevi, freckles, previous severe sunburn, any other skin cancer, or some form of immunosuppression. (I would add Scotch-Irish ancestry, red or blond hair, and hypopigmentation of the skin, or albinism.) Since a large portion of the American public has one or more of these characteristics, one would expect to see suitable restrictions or warnings posted at tanning centers—or better, have them banned outright. But the sale of tanning lights is permitted to private individuals as well as to licensed and unlicensed tanning salons alike, much to the detriment of public health.

Treatments Worse Than Cures?

In light of the known carcinogenic and age-accelerating properties of UV light, it may come as some surprise that physicians still use UV radiation as part of therapy for diseases as diverse as psoriasis and acne. Previously, only broad-spectrum wavelengths of light were used to treat a plethora of skin diseases. Practitioners argue that we know that the cancer-causing properties of UV light are concentrated at the shorter-wavelength and hence more energetic end of the spectrum (at about 290 to 300 nanometers), while only therapeutic effects are generated between 310 and 315 nanometers, where UV-A begins.

It is true that light sources that focus their rays within this latter range have proven to be remarkably effective in treating early stages of psoriasis. The "magic" to this treatment consists of adding an extract of coal tar known as psoralen plus ultraviolet light in the A range (PUVA therapy). Animal research demonstrates clearly that PUVA by itself or with a minimal dose of UV-B is highly carcinogenic. Adding a small dose of UV-B exposure made tumors appear even earlier.[6]

Does this mean PUVA (which lacks UV-B) is safe? Unfortunately, the major "therapeutic" light source is two to three times more cancer producing in test animals than is the broad-band sources used earlier.[7] The counterargument, that less light is needed to achieve a therapeutic result, is hardly reassuring to the patient who faces a possible second bout of disfiguring and perhaps life-threatening cancer once their basic psoriatic skin disease is cured. Considering that many psoriasis patients previously received the more carcinogenic doses, any additional treatment is likely to be adding fuel to the fire. As discussed in chapter 6, it is hoped that newer, more physiological treatments for psoriasis that rely on vitamin D analogs will soon be generally available.

Mechanisms

How UV light produces skin cancer is still a mystery. But it is clear that at least two different effects are involved, one direct and one indirect. At one time it was thought entirely due to UV's ability to damage DNA. Skin cells are particularly vulnerable to mutation after even a single exposure to energy-intense wavelengths of UV light. These mutations set the stage for the loss of control that presages cancer when they damage specific genes that keep cells normal or allow cells to escape their normal growth constraints. Later, new mutations may occur that permit the cell to become fully autonomous and free living (as in the case of a cancer cell). Should that event occur, the last remaining defense of the skin is to call forth an immune response that will recognize and destroy the incipient cancer cell. Unfortunately, this second-line defense system itself is vulnerable to damage and destruction by UV light!

Immunosuppression

Once it became clear that cancer could be produced in experimental animals by exposing them to UV light, researchers wanted to understand the biology of the resulting tumors. A key question was whether or not UV-induced skin cancers were detectable by the body's immune system. Such control, provocatively called immunologic surveillance, was in 1959 hypothesized by Lewis Thomas to be operating in the body. The idea of immune surveillance posits the existence of a population of cells from the immune system that recirculates throughout the organism, migrating randomly through the body's tissues in search of the defective and antigenic cells that commonly precede the development of full-blown malignancy. In theory, should a neoantigenic cell be detected, these lymphocytes attack and destroy it before it progresses to a tumor.[8] In 1968, I was the first to demonstrate the existence of such immune surveillance against skin cancer induced by chemicals.[9]

Dr. Margaret Kripke, now at the Baylor College of Medicine in Houston, Texas, examined this question by studying the possibility that UV light–induced skin tumors were antigenic. To her amazement, they turned out to be even more immunologically provocative than were the skin tumors I had studied. If this was indeed the case, she wondered, then why did so many skin tumors arise after the skin is exposed to UV light? A clue came from chemically induced tumor immunology: chemicals induced antigenic tumors in inverse proportion to their ability to knock out the immune system. Could it be, Dr. Kripke hypothesized, that ultraviolet light might also be immune suppressing? It made sense. How else to explain the survival of tumors that were induced with UV light? Virtually all were highly antigenic and hence subject to rapid detection and elimination.

Using white mice, which lack the protective pigmentation of their more deeply colored peers, Kripke found that UV light did indeed knock down the immune system. Most interestingly, the UV effect was due in large part to UV vulnerability of the antigen-processing, phagocytic Langerhans cells. After just a few minutes' exposure, a few cells would die. Depending on the dose, after an hour of exposure to UV light, the entire population of Langerhans cells could be cleared out of an area of skin, leaving an immunologic wasteland. While no one yet knows for sure the biological significance of this decimation, it is almost certain that the loss of a front line of defense here plays a critical role in the generation of skin tumors.

It is now clear that even low doses of UV light modify the immune system in the skin in a process known as photoimmuno-suppression.[10] In addition to the Langerhans cells, UV light kills or inactivates the other key cells in the skin that must exist to permit the skin to participate in generating an effective immune response. By taking out the skin cells that present antigens to the immune system and by inducing the formation of a group of other cells that suppress the immune system, UV light gives the immunologic-surveillance capacity of the skin a double whammy.[11] Heavily UV-exposed animals can neither recognize nor reject implanted UV-B-induced tumors, nor can they develop traditional forms of immune response, such as contact hypersensitivity, which might aid and abet any therapeutic strategies aimed at controlling their own tumors. Additionally, UV-B-exposed mice are much more susceptible to infection with bacteria, yeasts, or fungi than are unexposed normal mice.

Of particular concern in this day of AIDS is the possibility that any additional immune suppression could enhance the already high risks of infection of AIDS patients with organisms like *Candida albicans*, a common and sometimes lethal pathogen. The experimental demonstration that UV can reduce natural resistance to Candida, putting immunosuppressed mice at risk for lethal infections, is thus a cause for concern.[12] At best this data, still unsupported by human studies, means that it may be unwise for AIDS patients to sunbathe. In my view, limiting solar exposure is an essential part of health care for AIDS patients.

A similar pattern exists for leprosy. UV exposure in experimental animals increases their susceptibility to leprosy.[13] It is tempting to speculate that natural overexposure to sunlight contributed to the spread of leprosy into Polynesia and other areas where a relative lack of melanin pigment put populations at risk to UV-induced immune suppression.

An Evolutionary Quandary

☙ Even when the body's immune system is relatively unaffected, it is now clear that the skin is generally rendered unresponsive to new antigens after UV exposure. What can explain this state of affairs? Given the universality of sunlight, this reaction makes sense only if there is some evolutionary *advantage* for persons to shut down their skin immunity, however transiently, when overexposed to solar radiation. One explanation is that this immunosuppressive reaction is adaptive in dampening what might otherwise be an extreme inflammatory reaction to sunlight exposure that would make sunburns even worse than they are. Another is that immune suppression prevents autoimmune reactions set in motion by misrecognition of solar-damaged sunburn cells.

Still another rationale for local cutaneous immunosuppression is that it is outdoors that the body most likely is exposed to sensitizing chemicals. If sunlight dampens the reaction to poison oak and ivy, it may be beneficial in reducing the severity of immunologically mediated damage. It is also more likely that insect stings will occur during the daylight hours than at night. A system that reduced the skin's reactivity to such insect poisons might make evolutionary sense, since sensitization and anaphylactic reactions to bee or wasp stings can be fatal.

If there is an evolutionary explanation for this phenomenon, one would expect to find people with varying degrees of susceptibility to UV-induced immune depression—and that indeed appears to be the case. More to the point, patients with conditions like xeroderma pigmentosum, who develop basal or squamous cell cancer or related conditions, are now known to have genes that render them extremely UV-susceptible. Xeroderma patients appear to lack the DNA repair enzymes most of the rest of us possess. And the relatives of such persons, who typically carry a single dose of the xeroderma gene, appear also to be vulnerable to UV light. At a minimum, this discovery should permit at-risk individuals to be screened for sunlight sensitivity and advised accordingly. Certainly, full-blown UV suppression is likely to put individuals at risk for certain infectious diseases, an idea explored at length in a recent review.[14]

Prevention and Repair

Readers need not be reminded that the basic formula for keeping skin healthy includes avoidance of sunlight or, at a minimum, the use of an effective sunscreen. Indeed, a whole subfraction of the cosmetics industry is devoted to nothing else. One estimate puts the sun-care market worldwide at $2 billion.[15]

Some effective blockers include sunscreens that contain chemicals that absorb UV light. Each sunscreen preparation is assigned a sun protective factor (SPF) number. This number tells you how many extra minutes of exposure your skin can endure before being reddened or damaged by UV light. Thus, if it takes ten minutes to cause sunburn in a certain tropical setting, a sunscreen with a designated SPF number of twenty will allow you to stay in the sun for two hundred minutes before an equal sunburn occurs.

Unfortunately, too many people believe erroneously that a sunscreen provides indefinite protection against solar damage. Of course, you should stop exposure *before* two hundred minutes when using sunscreen with the SPF factor of twenty in the circumstances just described. A startling recent finding in mice shows that sunscreens with a wide range of SPFs appear to fail to protect against UV-induced skin cancer. If true, this means that staying out longer because you are wearing sunscreen may be counterproductive. The most obvious answer to avoiding solar damage is simply to stay out of the sun—completely. Or, barring your willingness to spend your life as a troglodyte, the best response is to protect yourself from the sun as much as possible. As the Australians put it, "Cover up, lather up, and button up": wear a hat, put on sunscreen lotion, keep your body covered.

A new generation of cosmetics that produce a tan without sunlight may allow you to dispense with sunscreens altogether, but only if you stay out of the sun after using them. Among the newest are cosmetics that dye the skin a light brown color without stimulating melanin synthesis. On a more prosaic level, some sunless tanning lotions simply superficially stain the skin a light brown. One in particular that contains an FDA-approved colorless dye is called Summer Vacation. This and related skin products can simply be applied overnight to produce a beautiful tan, but scarcely a solar-protecting tan. Moisturizers are used with these tanning dyes to prevent the drying effect of many chemical products.

Uneven tanning can be bolstered with makeup products with reassuring names like Sunny Disposition and Pinch Your Cheeks, a gel blush that enhances the tanned look by providing color to uniformly brown cheeks. Ideally, these and related products may come into widespread use to provide a "normal" tan without the burden of hours spent under a blazing tropical sun and thereby prevent the damage produced by overexposure to sunlight. But ironically, these new cosmetics may encourage precisely those behaviors they were intended to avoid: chemically tanned sunbathers may think their artificial bronzing provides protection against sunburn. It will not. Unwary of the continuing solar threat, these "tan safe" beauties may actually overdose on UV rays in the mistaken belief that they cannot be hurt once "tan."

Why this continued warbling about tanning and SPFs? All of this *Sturm und Drang* about the sun is intended to persuade you, dear reader, to abhor the sun. If you do not avoid the outdoors totally—and that would be a mistaken overreaction—at least take your doses of UV light in moderation.

But beyond these preventive approaches, new developments in molecular biology offer some promise of repairing the damage caused by ultraviolet light. One genetic engineering firm, Applied Genetics, Inc., has developed a "morning after" cream that will use the now well-known property of the skin to permit the penetration of large molecules to deliver the replacement genes for those damaged by UV light.

Another approach is to provide the skin with a DNA repair kit that will permit it to restore the DNA damage produced by UV sunlight.[16] Still another approach capitalizes on the finding that plankton near the ocean's surface contain even better repair kits for DNA damage. Being at the closest interface to the sunlight penetrating the ocean, many species of plankton contain an enzyme that speeds the recovery of DNA damage. Encapsulated and delivered in a new sunscreen product called Ocean Secret Day Formula, this cream accelerates the rate of tanning by stimulating melanin synthesis. (A related product called Ocean Secret Night Formula contains a related packet of enzymes derived from plankton.)

For all of these hypermodern advances, it appears that the lowly aloe plant, the mainstay of health food advocates for decades, may be just as effective a protectant for UV damage as any of these genetically engineered products. In recent research, an extract of *Aloe barbadensis* (aloe gel) was found to prevent UV-induced suppression of the immune system in the skin. Both contact and delayed hypersensitivity responses that are normally destroyed by UV-radiation exposure were protected by aloe gel in test animals treated *after* their exposure to a sunlamp source of UV light.[17] This finding clearly implies that putting on a bit of aloe gel may be distinctly more beneficial than relying on sun lotions or burn creams.

Melanoma

Tragically, even with these new protectants, skin cancers occur after sunning. In fact, some new research suggests that while most sunscreens do protect against the most damaging, carcinogenic rays of the sun, they still allow UV light to make animals susceptible to the growth of melanoma tumor cells. As we saw, the implications of this research are disturbing: if sunscreens encourage people to stay out in the sun longer than they might otherwise have done, they may increase the risk of outgrowths of melanoma that might be lying dormant in the body.[18] A partial explanation is that the sunscreens, while protective against visible damage, do not fully protect against immune suppression, thereby allowing tumor cells to sneak through what may normally be an effective defense system.

This latter point is not to be taken lightly. Of all the cancers that are sun related, none is more deadly than melanoma. This tumor often appears years after first solar exposure and, as we saw, is responsible for a growing number of deaths, especially among young adults. In terms of inducing melanoma, the worst time to be exposed to the sun is in childhood.[19] In contrast with adult exposures, where single, extreme sunburn is the most dangerous, both short-term and long-term solar exposure when you are a child appear comparably dangerous for melanoma risk.[20] In 1995, melanoma was more common among persons aged twenty-five to twenty-nine in the United States than any other form of nonskin cancer.[21] While melanoma takes many forms, its most deadly variety is the kind that rapidly penetrates the upper layers of the skin. Once below the basal membrane that separates epidermis from dermis, melanoma cells commonly migrate widely, metastasizing to distant organs like the lungs and liver, making it an unusually aggressive tumor.

Observations

❦ The tardiness of health professionals in sounding the alarm about ultraviolet light is a measure of how reluctant the medical profession is to entertain and embrace what now appears to be an unwelcome but almost self-evident truth. The ability of UV light to produce skin cancer has been known for over a half century and UV's cell-killing ability—especially of vulnerable lymphocytes in tissue culture—for almost as long. Even though for almost twenty years anatomists had identified cells in the skin that looked as if they might have immunologic activity, no one put together the compelling evidence of the existence of an immunologic apparatus in the skin until Margaret Kripke began her UV light studies in earnest in the 1980s.

Then all of the pieces suddenly came together: as we have seen, with solar exposure, the skin is not only damaged, but its underlying immune capabilities are destroyed.[22] These abilities were discovered concurrently with the UV cancer experimentation, leading to the discovery of the existence of a local hypersensitivity reaction and of a rudimentary immune system within the skin itself. These holistic observations make it essential to take even more seriously the consequences of ozone depletion. Now, with the influx of still more UV light, it is clear that the risks extend well beyond additional skin cancers to include reduced resistance to infectious diseases.

The fact that we continue to tolerate excessive suntanning and tanning parlors and fail to protect our children from the sun is a reflection of our cultural obsession with "looking fit" and being more concerned about appearance than long-term well-being.

THIRTEEN

The Future

We now recognize the skin as an amazingly adaptive structure that serves us well under almost all conditions we encounter. If subjected to extremes of heat or cold, the skin has an underlayment of blood vessels that almost instantly expands or contracts to protect the body within against overheating or freezing. If bombarded by reasonable amounts of ultraviolet radiation from the sun, skin cells repair the damage to their DNA and increase the skin's pigment content, protecting it against the next exposure. When attacked by microbes, the acid mantle of the skin retards their growth, and its superficial layers increase their rate of sloughing, throwing off offending spores or germs with a veritable shower of dead cells. If the microbial invasion is more intense, the skin initiates a vigorous immune response of its own. When interlopers penetrate a breach in its surface, the skin initiates a process of inflammation to process antigens for a broader immunologic assault and to clear away invading organisms, particles, or dirt. In a few days or weeks, migrating cells seal the damage, and any damage is repaired by a remarkably efficient healing process.

One can almost hear Shakespeare extol its virtues.

Is the skin not a marvel of invention?
If broken, it heals itself. If torn, it repairs the rift. If
burned, it restores itself. If frozen, it rebounds anew.
In love, it radiates warmth and gladness. In offense, it
turns fiery red. And in sorrow, it becomes pallid and
ashen, a reminder of our mortality.

We now know that the skin is an organ in and of itself. Its
role as a critical covering for our bodies is better appreciated
than ever before. Burn victims who have lost more than 40 percent of their skin surface can now be temporarily covered by a
meshwork of donor human skin or even short-lived grafts of
pigskin and survive otherwise fatal injury. But in the future, an
even more lasting substitute will be critically needed. Two new
candidates are products of modern technology that employ artificial matrices to grow skin from stem cells taken from the
foreskin or umbilical cord of a newborn infant. Others still in
development will use epidermal cells on an artificial dermis.

One company, Advanced Tissue Sciences, first developed a
skin substitute in 1987. Called Dermagraft, this novel product
is derived from foreskin fibroblasts that are grown on a scaf-
folding of a special plasticlike membrane that provides a "foot-
ing" for the cells to seed onto and spread out. Currently, the
product is still experimental and is grown in a closed perfusion
chamber that allows it to be frozen and shipped in a single con-
tainer for subsequent use in covering ulcers.

A related product called Grafskin is intended for us in treating burns and chronic wounds. It was developed by Organo-
genesis, a company based in Canton, Massachusetts. Currently,
Grafskin is used primarily as an artificial skin that permits testing of cosmetics outside the body of an animal.[1]

On the therapeutic front, iatrogenic or doctor-generated
problems are not likely to fade quickly from the scene unless

we learn from the mistakes we have made in the past. The newest generation of therapies for skin lesions and unsightly blood vessels still relies on the use of external sources of radiation, only in new forms. Lasers are and will be used increasingly to treat a variety of cutaneous pigmented disorders. The theory of laser therapy is simple and elegant: By concentrating a highly specific wavelength of light on pigmented skin, selected absorbtion of light energy can assure rapid and selective destruction of the targeted tissue. For those skin lesions that are superficial and pigmented, laser therapy is dramatically effective. Amateur tattoos and black tattoos respond dramatically to laser ablation, clearing up completely after a single treatment. Multicolored tattoos require multiple treatments, since no single laser wavelength of light will eradicate the variegated pigments completely. Pigmented nevi, which can precede melanoma, particularly one called the nevus of Ota, in which melanocytes deep within the dermis around the eyes produce a blue-gray discoloration, can also be laser treated and cleared completely after several treatments. Café-au-lait spots, those tan-colored patches of skin often seen on the face, are effectively eradicated after just a few laser exposures.

In such therapy, it is well to keep in mind the adage championed by this book: Superficial changes in the skin often reflect deeper changes within. In the instance of café-au-lait spots, a dermatologist would need to remember that such lesions are often a cardinal sign of a genetic condition known as neurofibromatosis, associated with tumors that form deep within the nervous system.

While tattoos are properly regarded as external symbols of our self-image, naturally occurring skin lesions are often symbolic manifestations of internal disorder. If we treat skin disorders as if they are only superficial diseases rather than reflections of deep-seated problems that affect the body as a whole, many systemic problems will persist. In the past, when we have seen an external manifestation of chemical poisoning or other toxicity, we have been lulled into complacency by thinking that the skin problems were the sole health issue that needed attention. Conditions like chloracne, which were once interpreted as the singular and sole toxic response to polychlorinated biphenyls (PCBs) or dioxin, hopefully will come to be recognized as signals of the chemical poisoning that produces deeper dysfunction in hormonal control and immune function.[2] It is now clear that both PCBs and dioxin pose a major threat of immunotoxicity and carcinogenicity and carry hidden dangers as mimics of critical body hormones.

If the past is any indication, we will evolve away from broad-spectrum antibiotics such as tetracycline to control skin infections. We will no longer continue to treat skin diseases symptomatically with therapies like nonspecific corticosteroids or radiation. Diseases such as psoriasis will succumb to specific vaccines that reinforce skin immunity against yeasts or other microorganisms. Nontoxic chemicals that concentrate in the skin's surface layers will be discovered that further strengthen the skin's defenses against a hostile microbial world. And the "light" problem of skin—too much and you have skin cancer, too little and you have rickets—will be solved with a deeper appreciation of the nuances of solar radiation.

Yes, sunlight is a tonic for healthy skin. The skin must absorb *some* radiation in order to make vitamin D precursors. It is even likely that regular exposure to sunlight is necessary to assure optimal hormonal balance. But it is all too clear that too much sunlight produces cancer. In the past, these tumors, which included squamous cell carcinoma and basal cell cancer, were widely regarded as treatable nuisances that required a little surgery once you reached your fifties and sixties. Today, with the profound immune depression that accompanies

AIDS, it is clear that even minor skin tumors can be fatal. And tumors like melanoma, which also have a solar connection, are much more complex and difficult to treat. As a heterogeneous group of related tumors, control of most but not all skin cancers depends on the eternal vigilance of the immune system. And protecting the immune system requires avoiding excessive solar exposure.

Treatments for serious skin diseases like psoriasis must move away from light therapy that combines UV light with dangerous coal tar extracts and psoralen. Even now, new light sources are being isolated that concentrate their radiation to only a few angstroms (for instance, 310–330 nanometers) and thereby overcome the problems produced by highly energetic, broad-wavelength light sources.[3] New technologies will, it is hoped, avoid the tragedies of "successful" treatments that reduce suffering from one disease in the short run but generate new disease problems in the long run. Ideally, as with X rays, we will one day learn to eschew medical treatments that produce delayed damage to the skin.

We have long associated beauty and health with superficial wellness. We prize a bronzed, wrinkle-free skin as the sine qua non of a healthy physiognomy. To ensure these qualities, we have encouraged interventions such as tanning salons, which produce short-term gains at the expense of long-term damage to bodily health and well-being.

The history of skin cosmetology is a long and broken trail of vanity, illusion, and medical catastrophes. Hexachlorophene, for example, the antibioticlike antiseptic, is still permitted for use under prescription for treating acne, even after it produced an epidemic of brain damage in nursery children. Silicone and collagen injections in the skin have left some patients literally scarred for life.

Today, we understand the biology of the skin in intricate detail. We know which genes change when it becomes cancerous; the molecular structures of its basic components; and the genetic makeup of almost all of the inherited diseases that plague its organization. What we lack is a sophisticated understanding of how everything fits together. We still do not understand how the skin responds to sun-induced damage or how its newly discovered immune cells work together to defend the body. We do not know what determines which few cells within the skin go on to produce cancers while all the remainder stay healthy. Nor do we understand how our skin ages and what can be done to keep it young. Or, for that matter, why and if wrinkled, "old" skin is any less adaptive than its smoother, younger counterpart.

Yet we let a whole cosmetics industry dictate "proper" skin care while knowledgeable medical professionals privately dispute the utility of even the most basic nostrums. We permit plastic surgeons to set the norms for facial and bodily beauty and how that superficial beauty is to be preserved, belying their own adage that beauty is more than skin deep. We tolerate a remarkable degree of trial-and-error medicine when it comes to the skin, tacitly acknowledging that many of the ministrations of dermatologists are still based on anecdotal evidence.

Even where we have tried to control bona fide disease of the skin, we have all too often erred on the side of the "quick fix" at the expense of successful, long-term salvation. We have a long history of misguided treatments of skin disease, beginning with the use of X rays to treat scalp ringworm in children. The resulting exposures of the head and neck to radiation produced a generation of thyroid cancer and, later, brain tumors in the "cured" patients.

To a pathologist concerned about world ecology, the answer is prevention: first, protect the ozone layer, which shields the earth from the more energetic and hence more carcinogenic

UV rays. Second, assure that optimal UV protection is available cheaply and inexpensively to a large cross section of the at-risk population. This means developing hypoallergenic, cheap sunscreens. One new possibility is the development of an artificial human melanin through genetic engineering. Biotechnology production of this product, put into a suitable cream base, would be a seemingly ideal solution. A third line of defense would be systemic DNA repair–facilitating drugs or antioxidants that would protect the skin from further damage once sunlight exposure had occurred. Fourth, limit unnecessary exposure from tanning beds.[4]

Unfortunately, the growing epidemic of skin cancer in the United States has failed to ignite the intense prevention efforts here that are so commonplace in Australia. Even there, the numbers of skin cancer deaths appear to be mounting at a disturbing rate. In the most recent year where statistics were available (1989–1990), 115 deaths were recorded in the province of Victoria from squamous cell carcinoma, a usually treatable form of skin cancer. Even these statistics were flawed, overlooking an additional 31 cases and misdiagnosing 17 others.[5] According to Professor Robin Marks of the University of Melbourne, the proper response to the absolute epidemic of skin cancer in his country is to concentrate on physician education so that tumors may be detected earlier, at a treatable stage. But this emphasis appears wrongheaded in view of the fact that skin cancer is preventable. Primary prevention is most desirable.

Medicalization of what is essentially a problem in prevention is infuriating to former public health professionals like myself. Where is the outrage against the Northern Hemisphere's overproduction of chlorinated and fluorinated hydrocarbons, which have put Australians in harm's way by depleting the ozone layer?

Dermatology as a specialty of medicine could use an infusion of vision. Instead of concentrating solely on superficial problems such as fungal infections of nails or tattoos (which in a recent review constituted two-thirds of the "most important" problems of dermatology),[6] clinicians would do well to recognize the skin's role as the border between wellness and dysfunction. It may be time to recognize the skin as the first bastion of our immunologic defenses *and* as a cardinal indicator of diseases within the body. Dermatology deserves to be recognized for its central role in medicine.

As we've seen, in truth, our skin is a portal to the outer world, a thin veil through which many things penetrate all too easily. Through even the most healthy skin, we remain exquisitely vulnerable to particular environmental insults. Ultraviolet light, streptococcal bacteria, or chemicals like dioxins and PCBs all readily gain entry through this portal. Yet the AMA has only just concluded in 1995 that tanning booths allow much too much DNA-damaging ultraviolet light to enter the body (even UV-A), and the EPA has only recently recognized that many of the chemicals of greatest health concern are notorious for their ability to be absorbed rapidly through the skin.

Scientists, also, have only belatedly recognized the fact that our skin is remarkable for its selective permeability to certain gases and chemicals. Often, workers are separated from disaster by the thinnest of margins. NIOSH, the federal agency responsible for protecting workers against chemical insults, has developed new "skin notations" for some chemicals because they penetrate the intact skin so readily that doses sufficient to cause illness are possible under normal work conditions.

On the therapeutic front, skin permeability has proven a benefit for a limited number of chemicals. As we have seen, where the skin is thin (on the inner surface of the arm or behind the ear), small drug-bearing patches may be placed that will provide continuous low-level doses of chemicals as diverse as testosterone for treating male impotence and scopolamine for seasickness. Today, pharmaceutical manufacturers are capitalizing on this "newly" discovered phenomenon, even as its limitations become more widely recognized. Hosts of new chemicals, including hormones and antihypertensive agents, are currently being planned for transdermal delivery, even though tolerance remains a major problem that limits drug potency delivered through the skin. Nicotine patches will become the method of choice for smoking cessation and for treating ulcerative colitis. These developments echo an age-old fascination with the "magic" by which invisible agents were put into the body by shamans and traditional practitioners who applied remedies by rubbing the skin with herbal preparations or leaves from medicinal plants.

Within the next decade, artificial skin will be a reality. Skin will be the preferred portal for "injecting" drugs into the body, as new technologies for carrying large molecules across the "permeation barrier" of the stratum corneum are developed. New, exotic-sounding techniques of electroporation, phonophoresis, or ionophoresis, relying on electricity, sound, or ions, will be used to carry peptides and other drug molecules across the skin and into the body—without making a break.[7]

To think of the body's edge as mere integument, a passive covering for all that lies within, is to denigrate this masterful organ's central functions in maintaining health and wellness. In an age increasingly confronted by assaults to our surface, the skin serves as the thin line at our body's edge that takes the brunt of an increasingly hostile environment. The more we face external threats, the more we have to bolster this critical bastion. If we fail to prevent environmental depredations, the edge we hold in the continuing battle between sickness and wellness will be eroded.

Biologically, the skin transcends its function as an elastic membrane that bends and stretches with our bodily movements. It is the membrane that separates the living from the nonliving. It is essential to our survival. Without it, we would be helpless bags of water, bones, and chemicals, subject to dissipation into an inhospitable environment.

The skin is an invaluable asset for psychic as well as physical well-being. Cutaneous stimulation is critical to normal development. Without it, a child's development may be stunted or impaired. Unable to feel his skin, an obsessive patient may disfigure himself irrevocably. Desperately needing to belong, a teenager may tattoo or scar it indelibly. Despairing of self-worth, a woman may permit it to be injected or cut to shape her self-image. For better or worse, the skin has been made our emblem of self-identity.

The skin, then, is our boundary line between inner wellness and external danger, between psychic openness and closed armoring. It turns colors with our emotions, sheds and coarsens as we age, becomes cancerous or inflamed if abused by chemicals or radiation, and shrivels and dries out with neglect. A blemish or rash can reveal as much about our inner state of health or disease as does the expression on our face. When the skin suffers, so does the soul. Teenagers have been known to commit suicide out of despair over ever fixing their disfiguring acne.

It is no accident that skin cancer is a metaphor of our modern era. As we age, one in five Americans will get cancer, most of it cancer of the skin. The message appears simple: Without youthful skin we live in fear of our mortality. But in our vain attempts to make it more beautiful, we risk losing it altogether. "Saving your own skin" is much more than a cosmetic feat of plastic surgical legerdemain. It is essential for our wholeness and integrity in an increasingly polluted world.

Notes

1. Introduction to the Integument

1. For this and other facts, I am indebted to Henry E. Sigerist's *Primitive and Archaic Medicine* (New York: Oxford University Press, 1967).

2. A wide-ranging review of the impact of Greek systems of thought in medicine can be found in the collection of essays in Henry Sigerist's authoritative *On the History of Medicine* (New York: MD Publications, 1960), 63 ff.

3. Marie-Louise Johnson, "Skin Diseases," in *Cecil Textbook of Medicine* (Philadelphia: W. B. Saunders, 1985), 2227.

4. Anita Roddick, *The Body Shop Book* (New York: Dutton, 1994), 41.

2. At the Boundary of the Self

1. Personal communication, Gordon Smith, CMT, Gualala, California, 31 July 1995.

2. See M. S. Driscoll, M. J. Roth, J. M. Grant-Kels, and M. S. Hale, "Delusional Parasitosis: A Dermatologic, Psychiatric and Pharmacologic Approach," *Journal of the American Academy of Dermatology* 29 (1993): 1023–1033.

3. Ibid.

4. See M. Van Moffaert, "Psychodermatology: An Overview," *Psychotherapy and Psychosomatology* 58 (1992): 125–136.

5. Jeffrey P. Callen et al., *Dermatological Signs of Internal Disease*, 2nd ed. (Philadelphia: W. B. Saunders, 1994), 341.

6. Mary Madison, "Care That Gets Under the Skin," *San Francisco Chronicle*, 26 June 1995, A-13–14.

7. Eurydice, "Scar Lovers," *Spin*, August 1995, 60–66, 110.

8. Ibid.

9. See W. Westhoff, "A Psychosocial Study of Albinism in a Predominantly Mulatto Caribbean Community," *Psychology Reports* 73 (1993): 1007–1010.

10. Cited in M. Lappé, *Genetic Politics* (New York: Simon & Schuster, 1979), 51.

11. See Mary Tannen, "Made in the Shade," *New York Times Magazine*, 2 July 1995, 38.

3. Anatomy Lessons

1. See H. Tagami, "Quantitative Measurements of Water Concentration of the Stratum Corneum in Vivo by High Frequency Current," *Acta Dermatological Venerologica Supplement* 185 (1994): 29–33.

2. H. Varendi, R. H. Porter, and J. Winberg, "Does the Newborn Baby Find the Nipple by Smell?" *Lancet* 344 (1994): 989–990.

3. See H. E. Evans et al., "Factors Influencing the Establishment of the Neonatal Bacterial Flora: The Role of Host Factors," *Archives of Environmental Health* 21 (1970): 514–519.

4. See D. A. Goldmann et al., "Bacterial Colonization of Neonates Admitted to an Intensive Care Environment," *Journal of Pediatrics* 93 (1978): 288–293.

5. R. E. Billingham and W. K. Silvers, "Studies on the Conservation of Epidermal Specificities of Skin and Certain Mucosas in Adult Animals," *Journal of Experimental Medicine* 125 (1967): 429–446.

4. Form and Function

1. See Maria Sibilia and E. F. Wagner, "Strain-Dependent Epithelial Defects in Mice Lacking the EGF Receptor," *Science* 269 (1995): 234–237.

2. The specific mutations are described in Dennis Roop, "Defects in the Barrier," *Science* 267 (1995): 474–475.

3. N. Scott Adzick and H. Peter Lorenz, "Cells, Matrix, Growth Factors, and the Surgeon," *Annals of Surgery* 220 (1994): 10–18.

4. See E. C. Leroy, "The Spectrum of Scleroderma," in S. A. Paget and T. R. Fields, eds., *Rheumatic Disorders* (Boston: Andover Medical Publishers, 1992), 173–183.

5. Modified from Table 11-2 in Leroy, 178.

6. Peter J. Lynch, *Dermatology*, 3rd ed. (Philadelphia: Williams and Wilkins, 1994), 3.

7. See Richard Nathan, "Archaic Leprosy Law Under Attack," *Nature Medicine* 1 (1995): 617.

8. J. L. Wemeau, "Calciotropic Hormones and Ageing," *Hormone Research* 43 (1995): 76–79.

5. Barrier or Sieve?

1. See Dennis Roop, "Defects in the Barrier," *Science* 267 (1995): 474–476.

2. B. Forslind, "A Domain Mosaic Model of the Skin Barrier," *Acta Dermatologica Venereologica* 74 (1994): 1–6.

3. Walter B. Shelley and E. Dorinda Shelley, *CMD: A Century of International Dermatological Congresses* (Park Ridge, N.J.: Parthenon Publishing, 1992), 53.

4. See T. F. Fischer, "Lindane Toxicity in a 214-Year-Old Woman," *Annals of Emergency Medicine* 24 (1994): 972–974.

5. See R. D. Kimbrough, "Review of the Toxicity of Hexachlorophene," *Archives of Environmental Health* 23 (1971): 119–122.

6. See especially Henry E. Sigerist's *Primitive and Archaic Medicine* (New York: Oxford University Press, 1967), 483 ff.

7. R. Garnier, D. Chataigner, M. L. Efthymious, I. Moraillon, and F. Bramary, "Paraquat Poisoning by Skin Absorption: Report of Two Cases," *Veterinary and Human Toxicology* 36 (1994): 313–315.

8. See R. A. Fenske, S. W. Horstman, and R. K. Bentley, "Assessment of Dermal Exposure to Chlorophenols in Timber Mills," *Applied Industrial Hygiene* 2 (1987): 143–147.

9. See P. G. Jorens and P. J. Schepens, "Human Pentachlorophenol Poisoning," *Human Experimental Toxicology* 12 (1993): 479–495.

10. See R. Stephens, A. Spurgeon, I. A. Calvert, et al., "Neuropsychological Effects of Long-Term Exposure to Organophosphate in Sheep Dip," *Lancet* 345 (1995): 1,135–1,138.

11. Reviewed in J. Raloff, "Swimmers May Get Hefty Chloroform Dose," *Science News*, 7 January 1995, 5.

12. H. I. Maibach and D. M. Anjo, "Percutaneous Penetration of Benzene and Benzene Contained in Solvents Used in the Rubber Industry," *Archives of Environmental Health* 36 (1981): 256–260.

13. See J. Hanke, T. Dutkiewica, and J. Piotrowski, "The Absorption of Benzene Throughout the Skin in Man," *Medicale Practicalsky* 12 (1961): 413–426.

14. See EPA, "Dermal Exposure Assessment: Principles and Applications," Interim Report No. EPA/600/8-91/001B. Office of Research and Development, Environmental Protection Agency, Washington, D.C., 1992.

15. Reported by R. A. House, G. M. Liss, and M. C. Wills, "Peripheral Sensory Neuropathy Associated with 1,1,1 Trichloroethane," *Archives of Environmental Health* 49 (1994): 196–199.

16. See Vera Fiserova-Bergerova, "Relevance of Occupational Skin Exposure," *Annals of Occupational Hygiene* 37 (1993): 673–685.

17. See D. R. Mattie, J. H. Brabau, and J. N. McDougal, "Significance of the Dermal Route of Exposure to Risk Assessment," *Risk Analysis* 14 (1994): 277–284.

18. The rate of absorption obeys Fick's law that relates diffusion speed to such factors as time, temperature, molecular size, and distance.

19. See H. L. Judd, "Transdermal Estradiol: A Potentially Improved Method of Hormone Replacement," *Journal of Reproductive Medicine* 39 (1994): 343–352.

20. See D. A. Barrett and N. Rutter, "Transdermal Delivery and the Premature Neonate," *Critical Reviews in Therapeutic Drug Carrier Systems* 11 (1994): 1–30.

21. See T. Iwasaki, T. Hamano, K. Aizawa, et al., "A Case of Pulmonary Amyloidosis Associated with Multiple Myeloma Successfully Treated with Dimethyl Sulfoxide," *Acta Haematologica* 91 (1994): 91–94.

22. See U. Thadani and R. J. Lipicky, "Ointments and Transdermal Nitroglycerin Patches for Stable Angina Pectoris," *Cardiovascular Drugs and Therapy* 8 (1994): 625–633.

23. This point is discussed in E. R. Cooper, "Vehicle Effects on Skin Penetration," in R. L. Bronaugh and H. I. Maibach, eds., *Percutaneous Absorption: Mechanisms-Methodology-Drug Delivery* (New York: Marcel Dekker, 1990), 525–530.

24. See G. R. Tom and M. Premer, "Hydrocortisone Cream in Clonidine Patch Dermatitis," *Annals of Pharmacotherapeutics* 28 (1994): 889–890.

6. Diseases of the Skin: A Short History

1. Ralph L. Thompson, *Glimpses of Medical Europe* (London: Butterworth, 1908).

2. This and other facts are documented in Walter B. Shelley and E. Dorinda Shelley, *A Century of International Dermatological Congresses* (Park Ridge, N.J.: Parthenon Publishing, 1992).

3. These observations were included in the firsthand notes of an attendee at the 1972 International Dermatology Conference held in Vienna. See Shelley and Shelley, 65.

4. The precise prevalence estimates as of 1985 were 0.69 percent for atopic dermatitis; 0.55 percent for psoriasis; and 0.49 percent for vitiligo.

5. The association of alcohol and psoriasis was first reported in 1994 (K. Poikolainen, T. Reunala, and J. Karvonen, "Smoking, Alcohol and Life Events Related to Psoriasis among Women," *British Journal of Dermatology* 130 [1994]: 473–477). See the discussion in the "Letters to the Editor" sec-

tion: D. A. Buckley and S. Rogers; and response by Malcolm W. Greaves, and Gerald D. Weinstein, "Treatment of Psoriasis," *New England Journal of Medicine* 333 (1995): 258–259.

6. This point is underscored in an excellent contemporary review by Malcolm W. Greaves and Gerald D. Weinstein, "Treatment of Psoriasis," *New England Journal of Medicine* 332 (1995): 581–588.

7. See B. S. Baker, A. F. Swain, H. Valdimarsson, and L. Fry, "T-cell Subpopulations in the Blood and Skin of Patients with Psoriasis," *British Journal of Dermatology* 110 (1984): 37–44.

8. E. William Rosenberg, Patricia W. Noah, and Robert B. Skinner, Jr., "Psoriasis Is a Visible Manifestation of the Skin's Defense Against Microorganisms," *Journal of Dermatology* 21 (1994): 375–381.

9. P. G. Sohnle and B. L. Hahn, "Epidermal Proliferation and the Neutrophilic Infiltrates of Experimental Cutaneous Candidiasis in Mice," *Archives of Dermatological Research* 281 (1989): 279–283.

10. Ibid.

11. See Greaves and Weinstein, 581–588.

12. See Jeffrey S. Dover and Kenneth A. Arndt, "Dermatology," *Journal of the American Medical Association* 273 (1995): 1668–1670.

13. See I. A. Pion, K. L. Koenig, and H. W. Lim, *Dermatology and Surgery* 21 (1995): 227–231.

14. The relevant studies are tabulated in a recent review by K. U. Schallreuter, R. Lemke, O. Brandt, et al., "Vitiligo and Other Diseases: Coexistence or True Association?" *Dermatology* 188 (1994): 269–275.

15. P. P. Majumder, J. J. Nordlund, and S. K. Nath, "Pattern of Familial Aggregation of Vitiligo," *Archives of Dermatology* 129 (1993): 994–998.

16. K. U. Schallreuter and J. Berger, "Vitiligo and Cutaneous Melanoma: A Case Study," *Dermatologica* 183 (1991): 239–246.

17. Schallreuter, Lemke, Brandt, et al., 269–275.

18. See Swapan K. Nath, Partha P. Majumder, and James J. Nordlund, "Genetic Epidemiology of Vitiligo: Multilocus Recessivity Cross-Validated," *American Journal of Human Genetics* 55 (1994): 981–990.

19. See Marie-Louise Johnson, "Skin Diseases," in *Cecil Textbook of Medicine* (Philadelphia: W. B. Saunders, 1985), 2243.

20. See W. S. Dai, J. M. LaBraico, and R. S. Stern, "Epidemiology of Isotretinoin Exposure During Pregnancy," *Journal of the American Academy of Dermatology* 26 (1992): 599–600.

21. A. A. Mitchell, C. M. Van Bennekom, and C. Louik, "A Pregnancy-Prevention Program in Women of Childbearing Age Receiving Isotretinoin," *New England Journal of Medicine* 333 (1995): 101–106.

22. J. L. Mills, "Protecting the Embryo from X-Rated Drugs," *New England Journal of Medicine* 333 (1995): 124–125.

23. See A. Coon, ed., *The Chirurgical Works of Percival Pott, F.R.S. and Surgeon to St. Bartholomew's Hospital*, vol. 3 (London: Lowden, Johnson, Bobinson, Caddle, Evans, Fox, Dew & Haven, 1783).

24. See K. Yamigawa, *Collected Papers on Artificial Production of Cancer* (Tokyo: Maruzen Co. Ltd., 1965).

25. R. L. Bronaugh, S. W. Collier, S. E. Macpherson, and M. E. Kraeling, "Influence of Metabolism in Skin on Dosimetry after Topical Exposure," *Environmental Health Perspectives* 102 (1994): 71–72.

26. See S. S. Devesa, W. J. Blot, B. J. Stone, et al., "Recent Cancer Trends in the United States," *Journal of the National Cancer Institute* 87 (1995): 175–182.

27. Ibid., Table 1, 176.

28. See A. G. Glass and R. N. Hoover, "The Emerging Epidemic of Melanoma and Squamous Cell Skin Cancer," *Journal of the American Medical Association* 262 (1989): 2097–2100.

7. Bolstering Skin Defenses

1. See R. L. Bronaugh, S. W. Collier, S. E. Macpherson, and M. E. Kraeling, "Influence of Metabolism in Skin on Dosimetry after Topical Exposure," *Environmental Health Perspectives* (supp.) 11 (1994): 71–74.

2. See G. L. Sussman and D. H. Beezhold, "Allergy to Latex Rubber," *Annals of Internal Medicine* 122 (1995): 43–46.

3. Cited in Albert Rosenfeld, "Some of a Body's Crucial Functions Are Only Skin Deep," *The Smithsonian* (May 1988): 159–180.

4. See D. Y. M. Leung, "The Immunologic Basis of Atopic Dermatitis," *Clinical Reviews in Allergy* 11 (1993): 447–469.

5. J. W. Streilein, "Skin Associated Lymphoid Tissue," chapter 2, in D. A. Norris, ed., *Immune Mechanisms of Cutaneous Disease* (New York: Marcel Dekker, 1989), 73–95.

6. See Elisabeth Payer, Adeheid Elbe, and Georg Stingl, "Epidermal T Lymphocytes—Ontogeny, Features, and Function," *Springer Seminars in Immunopathology* 13 (1992): 315–331.

7. See E. Tschachler, G. Schuler, J. Hutterer, H. Leibel, et al., "Expression of Thy-1 Antigen by Murine Epidermal Cells," *Journal of Investigative Dermatology* 81 (1983): 282–285; and P. R. Bergstresser, R. E. Tigelar, J. H. Dees, and J. W. Streilein, "Thy-1 Antigen-Bearing Dendritic Cells Populate Murine Epidermis," *Journal of Investigative Dermatology* 81 (1983): 286–294.

8. See J. A. Hill, K. Polgar, and D. J. Anderson, "T-Helper 1 Type Immunity Trophoblast in Women with Recurrent Spontaneous Abortion," *Journal of the American Medical Association* 273 (1995): 1933–1936.

9. See J. K. Salmon, C. K. Armstrong, and J. C. Ansel, "The Skin as an Immune Organ," *Western Journal of Medicine* 160 (1994): 146–152.

10. See especially the minireview by Lajos Kemény, Thomas Ruzicka, Attila Dobozy, and Günter Michel, "Role of Interleukin-8 Receptor in Skin," *International Archives of Allergy and Immunology* 104 (1944): 317–322.

11. An excellent review is available in Salmon, Armstrong, and Ansel.

12. G. Stingl, E. Tschachler, V. Groh, and K. Wolff, "The Immune Functions of Epidermal Cells, chapter 1, in D. A. Norris, ed., *Immune Mechanisms of Cutaneous Disease* (New York: Marcel Dekker, 1989), 3–72.

13. See K. Wolff and G. Stingl, "The Langerhans Cell," *Journal of Investigative Dermatology* 80 (1983): 17S–21S.

14. See C. Ezzell, "Tissue Engineering and the Human Body Shop: Designing 'Bioartificial' Organs," *Journal of NIH Research* 7 (1995): 49–52.

15. L. Blohme and O. Larko, "Premalignant and Malignant Skin Lesions in Renal Transplant Patients," *Transplantation* 37 (1984): 165–167.

16. Gaston N. King, Claire M. Healy, Mary T. Glover, et al., "Increased Prevalence of Dysplastic and Malignant Lip Lesions in Renal-Transplant Recipients," *New England Journal of Medicine* 332 (1995): 1952–1957.

17. See, for example, P. M. Collier and F. Wojnarowska, "Drug-Induced Linear Immunoglobulin A Disease," *Clinical Dermatology* 11 (1993): 529–533.

18. See D. Y. M. Leung, "Role of IgE in Atopic Dermatitis," *Current Opinion in Immunology* 5 (1993): 856–962.

19. See the review by C. Dezutter-Dambutant and D. Schmitt, "Epidermal Langerhans Cells and HIV-1 Infection," *Immunology Letters* 39 (1993): 33–37.

8. Hypersensitivity

1. Adapted from Harvey Rotstein, *Principles and Practice of Dermatology*, 3rd ed. (Boston: Butterworth-Heinemann, 1993), 27.

2. See C. G. Webster and J. W. Burnett, "Gold Dermatitis," *Cutis* 54 (1994): 25–28.

3. From figures reported in "FDA Committee Urges Stronger Warnings on Searle's Maxaquin," *SCRIP* 11 (1993): 32–36.

4. This issue is discussed at length in a review article by Satoshi Takayama, Masaakik Hirohashi, Michiyuki Kato, and Hiroyasu Shimada, "Toxicity of Quinolone Antimicrobial Agents," *Journal of Toxicology and Environmental Health* 45 (1995): 1–45.

5. See Leonard Hayflick's *How and Why We Age* (New York: Ballantine Books, 1994), 173.

6. See discussion in B. R. Krafchik, "The Use of Topical Steroids in Children," *Seminars in Dermatology* 14 (1995): 70–74.

9. Skin Signs of Illness

1. Marie-Louise Johnson, "Skin Diseases," in *Cecil Textbook of Medicine* (Philadelphia: W. B. Saunders, 1985), 2227.

2. These conditions and the diagnostic system of Chinese medicine more generally are described authoritatively in H. Beinfield and E. Korngold, *Between Heaven and Earth: A Guide to Chinese Medicine* (New York: Ballantine Books, 1991).

3. Dana Ullman, *The Consumer's Guide to Homeopathy* (Los Angeles: Tarcher/Perigee, 1996), 88.

4. See Jeffrey P. Callen et al., eds., *Dermatological Signs of Internal Disease*, 2nd ed. (Philadelphia: W. B. Saunders, 1994).

5. These and other symptom complexes are described by R. A. Watts and D. G. I. Scott, "Rashes and Vasculitis," *British Medical Journal* 310 (1995): 1128–1132.

6. Walter B. Shelley and E. Dorinda Shelley, *CMD: A Century of International Dermatological Congresses* (Park Ridge, N.J.: Parthenon Publishing, 1992), 21.

7. J. P. Callen, "Lupus Erythematosus," in Jeffrey P. Callen et al., eds. *Dermatological Signs of Internal Disease* (Philadelphia: W. B. Saunders, 1994), 3–12.

8. See D. Y. M. Leung, "The Immunologic Basis of Atopic Dermatitis," *Clinical Reviews in Allergy* 11 (1993): 447–469.

10. The Silicone Story

1. This point and other aspects of historical interest are taken from Pam Hait's "History of the American Society of Plastic and Reconstructive Surgery," published as a supplement to the September 1994 issue of *Plastic and Reconstructive Surgery*.

2. This impression was reported in a paper to the Society of Plastic and Reconstructive Surgeons in 1935 by New Orleans surgeon Robert Ryan.

3. This language appears in the original submission to the FDA on Form FD 1571, dated June 8, 1965, and titled "Dow Corning MDX 4-4011 Medical Fluid: 100 Centistokes and 12,500 Centistokes Viscosity. (For Tissue Augmentation by Injection Except for Mammary Area)."

4. Submission for investigational exemption for injectable silicones, Dow Corning to the FDA, dated June 8, 1965, p. 5.

5. See especially p. 8 of the IND submitted on June 8, 1965, by Dow Corning to the FDA for an exemption to use liquid silicone injections in people.

6. Ibid., p. 11.

7. Ibid.

8. Letter from Ralph Blocksma to Dow Corning of August 22, 1974.

9. See L. H. Winer, T. H. Sternberg, R. Lehman, and F. L. Ashley, "Tissue Reactions to Injections to Injected Silicone Liquids—A Report of Three Cases," *Archives of Dermatology* 90 (1964): 588–593.

10. This work was publicly reported by Dow Corning employees Silas Braley and Gordon Robertson in *Medical Engineering* in 1973. The internal document with the raw data is "Two-Year Studies with Miniature Silastic Mammary Implants TX-202A and TX-202B in Dogs," April 20, 1970.

11. B. Ellenbogen, R. Ellenbogen, and L. Ruben, "Injectable Fluid Silicone Therapy: Human Morbidity and Mortality," *Journal of the American Medical Association* 234 (1975): 308–312.

12. J. Chastre, F. Basset, F. Viau, et al., "Acute Pneumonitis after Subcutaneous Injections of Silicone in Transsexual Males," *New England Journal of Medicine* 308 (1983): 764–767.

11. Cosmetology

1. See Marc Lappé, *When Antibiotics Fail*, rev. ed. (Berkeley, Calif.: North Atlantic Books, 1995).

2. I am indebted to the Body Shop for these examples, in Anita Roddick, *The Body Shop Book* (New York: Dutton, 1994).

3. See R. F. Wehr and L. Krochmal, "Considerations in Selecting a Moisturizer," *Cutis* 39 (1987): 512–518.

4. J. M. Garden and R. K. Freinkel, "Systemic Absorption of Topical Steroids," *Dermatology* 122 (1986): 1007–1012.

5. See A. Dooms-Goossens, "Cosmetics as Causes of Allergic Contact Dermatitis," *Cutis* 52 (1993): 316–320.

6. Leonard Hayflick, *How and Why We Age* (New York: Ballantine Books, 1994), 111.

7. Cited by Hayflick, 170.

8. Ibid., 170.

9. Virginia L. Emster, Deborah Grady, Rei Milke, et al., "Facial Wrinkling in Men and Women, by Smoking Status," *American Journal of Public Health* 85 (1995): 78–82.

10. See I. Joffe, "Cigarette Smoking and Facial Wrinkling," *Annals of Internal Medicine* 115 (1991): 659, (letter).

12. The UV Story

1. These historical trends are cited in Anita Roddick, *The Body Shop Book* (New York: Dutton, 1994).

2. The UV wavelengths are broken into three main groups from longest to shortest: UV-A, UV-B, and UV-C. UV-A ranges from 320 to 400 nanometers. UV-B, the most damaging, is from 290 to 320 nanometers. UV-C, at 260 to 290 nanometers, is even more energetic and harmful and rarely reaches the earth's surface.

3. E. L. Speight, M. G. Dahl, and P. M. Farr, "Actinic Keratosis Induced by Use of Sunbed," *British Medical Journal* 308 (1994): 415.

4. Leonard Hayflick, *How and Why We Age* (New York: Ballantine Books, 1995).

5. L. R. Lever and C. M. Lawrence, "Nonmelanoma Skin Cancer Associated with Use of a Tanning Bed," *New England Journal of Medicine* 332 (1995): 1450–1451.

6. See R. D. Granstein, W. L. Morison, and M. L. Kripke, "Carcinogenicity of Combined Ultraviolet B Radiation and Psoralen Plus Ultraviolet A Radiation Treatment of Mice," *Photodermatology, Photoimmunology and Photomedicine* 9 (1992–1993): 198–202.

7. Described in Antony R. Young, "Carcinogenicity of UV-B Phototherapy Assessed," *Lancet* 345 (1995): 1431–1432.

8. This model has recently been reviewed in the special case of UV cancer: J. W. Streilein, J. R. Taylor, V. Vincek, et al., "Immune Surveillance and Sunlight-Induced Skin Cancer," *Immunology Today* 15 (1994): 174–179.

9. See M. Lappé, "Evidence for the Antigenicity of Papillomas Induced by 3-Methylcholanthrene," *Journal of the National Cancer Institute* 40 (1968): 823–846.

10. A recent review discusses the technical elements of this process: P. D. Cruz, Jr., "Ultraviolet B (UV-B)-Induced Immunosuppression: Biologic, Cellular and Molecular Effects," *Advances in Dermatology* 9 (1994): 79–94.

11. These effects and their experimental basis are summarized in Streilein, Taylor, Vincek, et al., 174–179.

12. See Y. M. Denkins and M. L. Kripke, "Effect of UV Irradiation on Lethal Infection of Mice with *Candida albicans*," *Photochemistry and Photobiology* 57 (1993): 266–271.

13. See A. Jeevan, K. Gilliam, H. Heard, and M. L. Kripke, "*Mycobacterium lepaemurium* Infection in Mice," *Experimental Dermatology* 1 (1992): 152–160.

14. See B. J. Vermeer and M. Hurks, "The Clinical Relevance of Immunosuppression by UV Irradiation," *Journal of Photochemistry and Photobiology*, series B 24 (1994): 149–153.

15. See Carol Potera, "Morning-After Cream Might Lighten Sun's Darker Side," *Genetic Engineering News*, 15 June 1995, 1, 14.

16. See P. Wolf, P. Cox, D. B. Yarosh, and M. L. Kripke, "Sunscreens and T4N5 Differ in Their Ability to Protect against UV-Induced Sunburn Cell Formation, Alterations of Dendritic Epidermal Cells and Local Suppression of Contact Hypersensitivity," *Journal of Investigative Dermatology* 104 (1995): 287–292.

17. F. M. Strickland, R. P. Pelley, and M. L. Kripke, "Prevention of Ultraviolet Radiation-Induced Suppression of Contact and Delayed Hypersensitivity by *Aloe barbadensis* Gel Extract," *Journal of Investigative Dermatology* 102 (1994): 197–204.

18. P. Wolf, C. K. Donawho, and M. L. Kripke, "Effect of Sunscreens on UV Radiation–Induced Enhancement of Melanoma Growth in Mice," *Journal of the National Cancer Institute* 86 (1994): 99–105.

19. See H. K. Koh, "Cutaneous Melanoma," *New England Journal of Medicine* 325 (1991): 171–182; and P. I. Ceballos, R. Ruiz-Maldonado, and M. C. Mihm, Jr., "Melanoma in Children," *New England Journal of Medicine* 332 (1995): 656–662.

20. S. L. Harrison, R. MacLennan, R. Speare, and I. Wronski, "Sun Exposure and Melanocytic Naevi in Young Australian Children," *Lancet* 344 (1994): 1529–1532.

21. Cited by Rex A. Amonette, M.D., president of the American Academy of Dermatology, *New York Times*, 1 July 1995, 14.

22. This story is told by M. L. Kripke in "Ultraviolet Radiation and Immunology: Something New under the Sun—Presidential Address," *Cancer Research* 54 (1994): 6102–6105.

13. The Future

1. These products are described in Jeffrey A. Hubbell and Robert Langer, "Tissue Engineering," *Chemical and Engineering News*, 13 March 1995, 42–53.

2. Judge Jack Weinstein dismissed most of the suit against Agent Orange by asserting that chloracne was the only condition ever associated with exposure to the dioxin (2,3,7 8 tetrachlorodibenzodioxin) that was the major contaminant of Agent Orange.

3. See B. L. Diffey, "Use of UV-A Sunbeds for Cosmetic Tanning," *British Journal of Dermatology* 115 (1986): 67–76.

4. "Health Issues of Ultraviolet 'A' Sunbeds Used for Cosmetic Purposes: A Statement by the International Non-Ionizing Radiation Committee of the International Radiation Protection Association," *Health Physics* 61 (1991): 285–288.

5. Peter Harrigan, "Skin Cancer in Australia," *Lancet* 345 (1995): 1,360.

6. See J. S. Dover and K. A. Arndt, "Dermatology," *Journal of the American Medical Association* 273 (1995): 1668–1670.

7. See I. Steinstrasser and H. P. Merkle, "Dermal Metabolism of Topically Applied Drugs: Pathways and Models Reconsidered," *Pharmacologica Acta Helvetica* 70 (1995): 3–24.

Index